To Lora with best regards,

Jim
11·18·93

Strategic Adaptation in the Health Professions

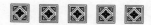

James W. Begun
Ronald C. Lippincott

    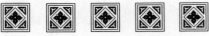

Strategic Adaptation in the Health Professions

*Meeting
the Challenges
of Change*

Jossey-Bass Publishers
San Francisco

Substantial discounts on bulk quantities of Jossey-Bass books are available to corporations, professional associations, and other organizations. For details and discount information, contact the special sales department at Jossey-Bass Inc., Publishers. (415) 433-1740; Fax (415) 433-0499.

For sales outside the United States, contact Maxwell Macmillan International Publishing Group, 866 Third Avenue, New York, New York 10022.

Manufactured in the United States of America

10% POST CONSUMER WASTE

The paper used in this book is acid-free and meets the State of California requirements for recycled paper (50 percent recycled waste, including 10 percent postconsumer waste), which are the strictest guidelines for recycled paper currently in use in the United States.

The ink in this book is either soy- or vegetable-based and during the printing process emits fewer than half the volatile organic compounds (VOCs) emitted by petroleum-based ink.

The epigraph at the beginning of the book is reprinted with permission from Freymann, J. G. "Medical Cost Containment: Preparing for the Year 2010." In J. D. McCue (ed.), *The Medical Cost-Containment Crisis: Fear, Opinions, and Facts.* Ann Arbor, Mich.: Health Administration Press, 1989.

Library of Congress Cataloging-in-Publication Data

Begun, James W.
    Strategic adaptation in the health professions : meeting the challenges of change / James W. Begun, Ronald C. Lippincott.
      p.   cm. — (The Jossey-Bass health series)
    Includes bibliographical references and index.
    ISBN 1-55542-582-8 (alk. paper)
    1. Medical personnel. 2. Medicine — Societies, etc. 3. Medicine — Practice. I. Lippincott, Ronald C., date. II. Title.
III. Series.
    [DNLM: 1. Health Personnel — organization & administration — United States. 2. Societies — organization & administration — United States. 3. Health Occupations — trends — United States.   W 21 B418s 1993]
    R728.B42 1993
    610'.6 — dc20
    DNLM/DLC
    for Library of Congress   93-13377
                                                    CIP

FIRST EDITION
HB Printing   10 9 8 7 6 5 4 3 2 1   *Code 9383*

The Jossey-Bass Health Series

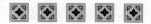

Contents

**Part Three: Profiles of
Diverse Health Professions**

Figures and Tables

Figures

Tables

Preface

Health professionals and their associations face an uncertain and complex work world today. The stable era of retrospective reimbursement, consumer acceptance of professional authority, and rigid definition of professional boundaries is gone. In its place is a more dynamic and contentious set of pressures—market competition among large delivery systems, persistent demands from consumers and third-party payers for relief from ever-increasing prices, and dissatisfaction with the inaccessibility of professional services to many who need them.

In this environment, the conventional strategies used to build the health professions are ineffective. New strategies, suited to contemporary conditions, are required. New attitudes and behavior on the part of practitioners and their associations are needed if the health professions are to continue to meet the goals of their members and those of society at large.

Audience

The purpose of *Strategic Adaptation in the Health Professions* is to help health professionals and those who work with them understand, predict, and shape their changing work world. The book

is meant to empower health professionals — to enhance their contributions to their associations and to society. Those who are
concerned about the direction of their profession, as well as
leaders of local, state, and national professional associations,
are an important audience of this book.

The book is directed also at educators of health professionals, due to their key role in shaping the coming generations
of health professionals, and the students who will make up those
generations. Health care managers and policy makers will gain
a greater appreciation for a basic (and frustrating) complexity
in their own work worlds: health care organizations and systems are very difficult to manage and regulate externally. This
is because those who deliver services belong to professions, and
professions have collective interests of their own. Finally, scholars
of the professions will be interested in the profession-building
strategies outlined here and the comparisons of different health
professions.

Overview of the Contents

The book is divided into three parts. Part One (Chapters One
and Two) gives the foundation for the book. Chapter One describes the challenging new environment faced by health professionals, contrasting it with the more benevolent environment
of the past. This shift has created a need for new strategies to
achieve adaptation. Chapter Two conveys the conceptual framework defining the major stakeholder relationships that professionals and their associations must manage. In this chapter we
conceptualize professions as loosely coupled communities of individuals and associations whose collective strategies can be plotted
and managed.

Part Two (Chapters Three through Seven) analyzes the
various strategies that health professions have used to pursue
the goals of legitimacy and market power and to manage their
internal dimensions. Throughout Part Two we contrast "conventional" strategies with "contemporary" strategies that are
better suited to the new environment. Chapter Three presents

strategies to achieve and maintain legitimacy. Next we consider strategies that relate to achieving market power—under the rubric of managing relationships with substitutes (Chapter Four), suppliers (Chapter Five), and buyers (Chapter Six). Chapter Five is shorter than the others owing to the lesser importance of supplier relationships in most professions. In Chapter Seven, we outline a series of internal organization and management issues faced by professional communities and discuss the conventional and contemporary strategies for addressing these issues.

Part Three (Chapter Eight) offers short analyses of five health professions to illustrate application of the strategic adaptation framework: medicine, optometry, registered nursing, physical therapy, and occupational therapy. Examples from other professions, such as pharmacy and health administration, are given throughout the book. The use of diverse examples should help members of specific professions to apply the framework to their own work. Moreover, application of the same framework across professions should help professionals to learn from the experiences of others.

In this book, we take seriously Eliot Freidson's observation (1989, p. 190) that professions are not just aggregates of individuals but "organic social entities." They are organized systems of people and associations including not just practitioners but also, at various times, teachers, researchers, administrators, and regulators. Our concept of the "professional community," therefore, is broader than most concepts of the profession. This book draws on material from organization theory, business strategy, and the sociology of the professions. In the lexicon of organization theory, the perspective is a "strategic choice" approach: the profession is viewed as a collective possessing the free will to choose among different strategies in order to adapt to change and even shape it.

We explore changes in the health care environment from the standpoint of the individual profession rather than the position of the policy maker, consumer, or evaluator. We assume that strategic adaptation of the professions is a valued outcome. Whether this is a widely shared assumption outside the professions depends on what professions do with their powers. In this regard, our perspective is one of "enlightened self-interest," which recognizes that professions seek self-interest, but within the context of society's constraints. We argue that long-term survival of the professions requires that they balance their own interests with those of their key stakeholders. Therefore, for example, economic self-interest is pursued within the context of society's expectations that economic power will not be abused and professions will serve public interests in order to maintain social legitimacy.

Our framework is intended to apply to all the health professions. The use of diverse professions in the anecdotes and case examples throughout the book is meant to stimulate comparative thought about these professions in contrast to the customary case studies of individual professions. We have also tried to avoid the customary emphasis on medicine. This is consequential not only due to the size and importance of the other health professions but to the growing challenges to medicine's historical domination of health care.

While much of the material in the book applies best to the clinical professions, we include examples from administrative professions, such as health care administration and medical record administration, as well. Administrative professions are facing the same general changes being experienced by clinical professions, although their relationships with external stakeholders differ in many ways.

Acknowledgments

Several friends and colleagues offered advice or encouragement at various points in the process of writing this book: Tom Barker, Roice Luke, Dennis Pointer, Scott Sullivan, Janet Watts, John Whitener, and Tom Wyman. The assistance and understanding of our editor, Rebecca McGovern, and Luana Morimoto of Jossey-Bass were quite heartening. Comments from three anonymous reviewers were eye-opening and stimulating. Lippincott's semester-long sabbatical from the University of Baltimore was instrumental in accomplishing this work.

Above all, we thank our parents and our immediate families — Suellen, Jean, Mitch, and Michael — whose nourishment of our daily lives both inspired us and helped us keep this undertaking in perspective.

August 1993

James W. Begun
Richmond, Virginia

Ronald C. Lippincott
Baltimore, Maryland

In memory of my brother, Martin
—James W. Begun

The Authors

James W. Begun is professor and director of doctoral studies in health services organization and research in the Department of Health Administration, Medical College of Virginia, Virginia Commonwealth University. He is a research associate of the Williamson Institute for Health Studies, Virginia Commonwealth University, and the Health Services Research Center, University of North Carolina. Begun received his B.A. degree (1972), summa cum laude, as well as his M.A. (1975) and Ph.D. (1977) degrees in sociology, from the University of North Carolina at Chapel Hill (UNC–CH). He has taught in the Department of Social and Administrative Medicine at UNC–CH and the School of Business and Public Administration at Cornell University.

Begun's research interests are in the areas of health occupations and professions, health policy, and health organization design. He is the author of numerous journal publications and book chapters on these topics, as well as *Professionalism and the Public Interest* (1981).

In 1986 Begun served as a visiting scholar at the Center for Health Services Education and Research, St. Louis University, and he was program chair and chair of the Health Care

Administration Division of the Academy of Management in 1987–88 and 1989–90. He served on the Dissertation Grants Review Committee of the Agency for Health Care Policy and Research and as a site visitor of the Accrediting Commission on Education for Health Services Administration. He has been an associate editor of the *Journal of Health and Social Behavior* and a guest editor of *Medical Care Review.* Currently he is on the editorial board of *Medical Care Review.* Begun also has served as a consultant to the U.S. Federal Trade Commission, the Virginia Board of Health Professions, the North Carolina Governmental Evaluation Commission, and several other public and private organizations.

Ronald C. Lippincott is associate professor in the Department of Government and Public Administration at the University of Baltimore. He received his B.S. degree (1969) in political science from Rutgers University, his M.R.P. degree (1971) in social policy planning from UNC–CH, and his Ph.D. degree (1981) in political science from UNC–CH.

Lippincott's primary research interests have been in the politics of health care, the sociology of occupations, organization theory, and state politics. His work has appeared in the *Journal of Health Politics, Policy and Law, Work and Occupations,* and *Policy Studies Journal.* In addition, he has coauthored (with James W. Begun) a chapter in *Strategic Management of Human Resources in Health Services Organizations* (1988) and has recently completed a chapter (with Larry Thomas) in *Interest Group Politics in the Northeast* (1993).

Strategic Adaptation in the Health Professions

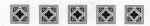

To those of us who grew up in the world of twentieth century medicine, the new millennium so close at hand is strange and frightening.

—John Gordon Freymann, MD

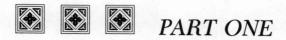

PART ONE

A Framework
for Strategic Adaptation

Chapter One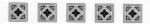

New Challenges
in the Health Professions

There is no doubt that the work world of health professionals
has changed dramatically in recent years. Whether these changes
are viewed with alarm, as in the case of the physician quoted
in the epigraph to the book, or with optimism, health professionals in the United States find themselves in a position of
greater uncertainty than ever before. For decades, the health
professions enjoyed the advantages of formidable governmental,
business, and public support. In no other sector of the economy were professionals so trusted to serve the public and so encouraged to incorporate the latest in new knowledge and technology in their work. To some extent this support is attributable
to the essential roles these professionals play in the drama of
life and death.

In recent years, however, health professionals have dis-
covered that the benevolence of their work world is eroding in
the face of growing concern over their responsiveness to public
needs. At the heart of this changing public view is the menac-
ing health care cost problem — a problem that is almost imper-
vious to control and comes at a time when economic restraint
has become the watchword of private industry and local, state,
and federal governments. Health professions have been identified

3

as a major source of the problems of access to health care and its growing cost.

Pressures to deliver more cost-effective, accessible services come from traditional sources — consumers, private employers, legislative bodies, and others who have historically been charged with responsibility for monitoring and financing the work of health professionals. But in addition, a new development is presenting an uncommon challenge. That new development is an increasingly unpredictable and turbulent marketplace for health care. Rivalry within and between professions has flourished, as large health care delivery organizations, potential substitute professions, and insurers have begun to challenge the status quo in the division of health care labor. Health professionals now often find themselves as adversaries, rather than allies, of health insurance companies and hospitals, both of which are struggling to retain market shares in the face of greater competition. Their world is increasingly populated by larger and more complex, vertically and horizontally integrated, business enterprises that are judged by their ability to compete in an economic marketplace. Most health professionals, in fact, work for these new players in the health care marketplace. Further uncertainties are introduced by new demands made by an aging and more health-conscious population, the seemingly intractable presence of a large number of uninsured or underinsured consumers, a persistent concern over rising malpractice costs and claims, and continuing disparities in accessibility to health services along racial and income lines.

It is in this context that health professionals, after years of relative insulation from external economic and political scrutiny, are more and more being treated like business inputs into the "product" called health care. Large health care corporations strive to routinize and "rationalize" professional work in order to manage it, and in this sense many health professions are undergoing a degree of "deprofessionalization." The growing complexity and change in this environment mean that professionals and their associations must reconsider their relationships with private third-party payers, hospitals, government agencies, the public, other professions, and even the members of their own professions. And this means that they and their professional associations must understand the strategies and strategic adaptation of their professions. *Strategies* are patterns in the goal-directed plans and activities of professionals and their associations that position the profession in relation to external demands. *Strategic adaptation* is the process whereby professions shift their strategies in response to new demands (Shortell, Morrison, and Friedman, 1990, pp. 27, 29).

To understand the need for strategic adaptation in the health professions requires an understanding of their changing environment. Toward that end, we first review indicators of the condition of these professions over the past several decades. Then, in more detail, we describe the growing uncertainty in the conditions affecting the health professions.

Expansion of the Health Professions

The health professions in the United States have shown remarkable vitality throughout the twentieth century. Rarely do these professions ever die a natural death; rarely, in fact, do they even contract in size. Of sixteen groups of practitioners traced by Aries and Kennedy (1986), all increased in numbers over the 1950–1980 period. Of the professions listed in Table 1.1 for which data are available, none declined in absolute numbers between 1950 and 1990, and none even decreased in numbers relative to the population. Many health professions, particularly the allied health professions, more than doubled their numbers per 100,000 population in the past two decades.

This century, particularly the period since World War II, has been truly remarkable in terms of this country's support of the establishment of new health professions and the continued success of old ones. As shown by the dates in Table 1.2, the oldest of the health professions in the United States (as indicated by the dates of formal organization of their primary professional association) are pharmacy, dentistry, and allopathic (conventional) medicine, all organized well before 1900. Around the turn of the century, the field of health professions became more crowded, as the original three were joined by registered nursing,

Table 1.1. Size of Selected Health Professions:
1950, 1970, and 1990.

Profession	Numbers in thousands			Numbers per 100,000 population		
	1950	1970	1990	1950	1970	1990
Administrators, health care	3	8	18	2	4	7
Administrators, long-term care	—	16	24	—	8	10
Chiropractors	13	14	45	9	7	18
Dental hygienists	7	40	81	5	20	32
Dental lab technicians	15	31	70	10	15	28
Dentists	79	102	149	52	50	60
Dietitians	—	17	67	—	8	27
Medical record administrators	—	10	18	—	5	7
Medical technologists	—	65	184	—	32	74
Nurse anesthetists	5	14	21	3	7	8
Nurse-midwives	—	1	4	—	1	2
Nurses, registered	335	750	1,627	218	364	651
Occupational therapists	3	6	34	2	3	14
Optometrists	15	18	26	10	9	10
Pharmacists	88	114	162	57	54	65
Physical therapists	5	30	71	3	15	28
Physician assistants	0	0.2	20	0	<1	8
Physicians — DOs	11	12	31	7	6	12
Physicians — MDs	209	311	537	134	149	215
Podiatrists	6	7	12	4	3	5
Psychologists	—	13	57	—	6	23
Radiologic service workers	—	87	122	—	42	49
Recreational therapists	—	6	35	—	3	14
Respiratory therapists	—	11	56	—	5	23
Social workers, medical	6	25	—	4	12	—
Speech-language pathologists and audiologists	—	19	85	—	9	34

Note: Dashes indicate data not available. Figures for 1990 are for the nearest available year. Nurse anesthetists and nurse-midwives are also included in the count of registered nurses. Health care administrators represent the count of active members of the American College of Healthcare Executives.

Source: Data from several sources. Primary sources include Aries and Kennedy, 1986; Institute of Medicine, 1989; Moscovice, 1984; U.S. Department of Health, Education, and Welfare, 1974; U.S. Department of Health and Human Services, 1980, 1988, 1992; and personal communications with professional associations.

optometry, osteopathy, podiatry, and psychology. Respiratory therapy, physician assisting, recreational therapy, denturism, certified nurse-midwifery, and long-term-care administration have largely developed since World War II, along with many smaller professions not listed in the table, such as technologists in the fields of diagnostic medical sonography, perfusion, and nuclear medicine.

As a result, the labor intensity of health care delivery has grown remarkably over the years. At the turn of the century, health workers comprised about 1 percent of the civilian labor force — about one-third of these were physicians; one-third were nurses, midwives, and attendants; and the remainder were veterinarians, pharmacists, dentists, and lens makers and grinders. The percentage of the labor force providing health care services climbed to about 2 percent by 1930 and 5 percent by 1970 and is expected to reach 10 percent by the year 2000 (Caress, 1976; U.S.Department of Commerce, 1990). Total health care workers were estimated by the federal government to include about 2.5 million in 1960 and 4 million in 1970 (U.S. Department of Health, Education, and Welfare, 1974). Another source reports some 4.2 million health services workers in 1970, 7.3 million in 1980, and 9.4 million in 1990 (Jonas, 1990, p. 53; U.S. Bureau of Labor Statistics, 1991, p. 199).

Many of the newer health occupations and professions are employed in hospitals. Between 1950 and 1990, the number of full-time employees per short-term hospital bed steadily climbed from 1.31 to 3.68 (American Hospital Association, 1991, p. 4). Compared to other nations, the United States generally has high ratios of health professionals to population and greater specialization within the health labor force. Osteopaths, podiatrists, and optometrists, for example, are not found in many other countries, nor are many of the specialized allied health professions (Jonas, 1990, p. 54). Indeed, the exact number of health occupations and professions in the United States is difficult to quantify. The job description manual of the American Society for Hospital Personnel Administration of the American Hospital Association provides detailed descriptions of 335

Table 1.2. Primary Professional Associations.

Profession	Primary Professional Association	Year Founded
Administrators, health care	American College of Healthcare Executives	1933
Administrators, long-term care	American College of Health Care Administrators	1962
Chiropractors	American Chiropractic Association	1930
Dental hygienists	American Dental Hygienists' Association	1923
Dentists	American Dental Association	1859
Denturists	National Denturist Association	1975
Dietitians	American Dietetic Association	1917
Medical record administrators	American Medical Record Association	1928
Medical technologists	American Society for Medical Technology	1932
Nurse anesthetists	American Association of Nurse Anesthetists	1931
Nurse-midwives	American College of Nurse-Midwives	1955
Nurses, registered	American Nurses' Association	1896
Occupational therapists	American Occupational Therapy Association	1917
Optometrists	American Optometric Association	1898
Pharmacists	American Pharmaceutical Association	1852
Physical therapists	American Physical Therapy Association	1921
Physician assistants	American Academy of Physician Assistants	1968
Physicians – DOs	American Osteopathic Association	1897
Physicians – MDs	American Medical Association	1847
Podiatrists	American Podiatric Medical Association	1912
Psychologists	American Psychological Association	1892
Radiologic technologists	American Society of Radiologic Technologists	1920
Recreational therapists	National Therapeutic Recreation Society	1966
Respiratory therapists	American Association for Respiratory Care	1947
Social workers, medical	National Association of Social Workers	1918[a]
Speech-language pathologists and audiologists	American Speech-Language-Hearing Association	1925

[a]Founding date is for the American Association of Hospital Workers, later renamed the American Association of Medical Social Workers, which merged with the National Association of Social Workers in 1955 (Burek, 1992; Hollis and Taylor, 1951).

Source: Backus, 1990.

different occupational roles within the hospital (American Society for Hospital Personnel Administration, 1985). A recent career guide lists 120 different careers in the health care field, from animal technician to ward clerk (Alperin and Rose, 1989), while a 1986 sourcebook on health occupations lists 121, from acupuncturist to veterinarian (National Commission for Health Certifying Agencies, 1986). The federal government listed 181 primary titles and 536 alternate titles for health occupations in 1977, a total of 717 different designations (U.S. Department of Health, Education, and Welfare, 1977b).

In addition to witnessing the growth of their professions, most health professionals have accrued job security, income, and prestige. These professionals in the past have not faced the specter of unemployment, displacement by machinery, or autocratic working conditions encountered by millions of workers. They have largely enjoyed steady employment, income growth, and respect from employers and society.

Historical Sources of the Benign Environment

The high survival rate of health professions and the steady patterns of growth in the number of professions and the supply of professionals reflect the fact that these professions have enjoyed a general environment that has been not only munificent but predictable. By general environment we mean conditions in the demographic, economic, cultural, governmental, and knowledge sectors of society that affect the work of health professionals.

The steady population growth of the United States, averaging 1.6 percent annually since 1950 (U.S. Bureau of the Census, 1991), has contributed to the stability of this environment. Per capita real disposable income has grown by at least 15 percent in each of the past four decades (U.S. Bureau of the Census, 1991, p. 434). The abundance of "customers" has kept to a minimum struggles over professional turf, since most health professions have had ample work for their members. Population growth continues to stimulate demand for their services, particularly those who serve the growing portion of the population that is over sixty-five years of age. Population growth will remain a major source of stability in the future.

Financial support for the work of the health professions has been steadily growing as well. The percentage of GDP devoted to health care in the United States climbed from 4.4 to 13.2 percent between 1950 and 1991 (Health Insurance Association of America, 1989; U.S. Department of Health and Human Services, 1993). Very few other economic sectors could have nurtured the growth and proliferation of professions to such an extent. The United States is by far the nation devoting the largest portion of its resources to health care (Schieber, Poullier, and Greenwald, 1992). Growth in payments for professional services has paralleled or exceeded growth in total health expenditures over the 1950–1990 time period (Levit, Lazenby, Letsch, and Cowan, 1991). Government policies directing resources to the health sector, such as the Medicare and Medicaid programs, contributed to this growth, as did the steady expansion of the American economy.

The federal government's benevolence toward the health sector, including health professionals, began in large part after World War II with the Hill-Burton Act to fund hospital construction and with development of the National Institutes of Health to fund the development of new knowledge. Significant federal aid for professional education began with the Health Professions Educational Assistance Act of 1963, which provided construction funds and operating support for medical, dental, pharmacy, podiatry, nursing, optometry, and public health schools, as well as loan and scholarship programs. Educational support for veterinary medicine and allied health professions soon followed. Implementation of the Medicare and Medicaid programs in 1965 acknowledged the tacit backing of federal and state government for the existing provider-dominated cost reimbursement system that financed, directly or indirectly, many health professional services. The 1968 Health Manpower Act extended and expanded federal largess to the health professions. Federal dollars flowing into the health professions have been credited with a major role in expanding the health worker pool from 2.5 million to 6 million workers, as well as promoting intricate specialization into different professions and specialties within professions (McTernan and Leiken, 1982). Moreover, the system's ability to absorb large numbers of new professionals has kept conflict within and among professions to a minimum.

The vast and expanding technology and knowledge base of health care delivery is another force that created pressures for a highly specialized division of labor and for a cadre of professionals educated in institutions of higher learning. Significant developments in new knowledge and technology have spawned new professions and enabled older ones to claim new tasks that are exciting, publicly legitimated, and financially rewarding to the provider. It has been estimated that over 60 percent of the real growth in the cost of medical care between 1950 and 1985 can be attributed to new technologies (Janeway, 1989). The federal government has been a supporter of this trend, funding some two-thirds of biomedical research and development, largely through the National Institutes of Health (Hillman, 1987). The government has generally ceded control over research to the scientific community, letting clinical and research professionals make funding decisions about research (Starr, 1982, p. 343).

This benign environment has been reinforced by the granting of professional self-regulation over entry to the profession and the conduct of practice. Legal control over entry and professional practice is mainly a function of state government, and requirements that health practitioners be licensed, certified, or registered are found throughout the states. Registration, the least restrictive form of regulation, usually takes the form of requiring individuals to file their name, address, and qualifications with a government agency before practicing the occupation. Under public certification, another form of regulation, the government grants title protection to persons meeting predetermined standards. Those without the title may perform the services but cannot use the title. Licensure, the strongest form of state government regulation, makes it illegal for a person to practice without first meeting standards imposed by the state (Council of State Governments, 1990). In 1990, some 115 different health occupations were licensed in at least one state, an additional 13 were certified in at least one state, and an additional 9 were registered in at least one state (Council of State Governments, 1990). Strong regulation, defined by licensure in at least forty states, extends to fifteen of the twenty-six professions listed earlier in Table 1.1.

Typically, the regulated professions are involved extensively in setting and enforcing entry and practice standards (Gross, 1984; Young, 1987). These structures ensure a degree of standardization and professional control over the number and type of people who practice a certain profession. They also create small cartels, whose members are better able to control competition among themselves and present a united front against external forces.

Another source of stability in the health professions' environment has been the relative concentration of control over the division of labor in two professions: medicine and dentistry. These two professions have carved out broad spheres of work that historically have constrained the ability of most other health professions to compete against medicine and dentistry. While the dominance of medicine and dentistry has not necessarily contributed to the welfare of the other health professions, the division of labor has protected the health professions from outright warfare over turf. Related professions were assigned tasks that physicians and dentists did not want to perform, and they were relegated to subordinate relationships to physicians and dentists. The subordinate legal status and narrow work domains meant that most health professions developed quite explicit relationships with other professions. In the medical care sector, Scott and Lammers (1985, p. 67) say that physicians have been able to provide "an important source of integration and coherence to the sector as a whole."

A final source of the benign environment has been public respect for science, for the sanctity of life, and for the persuit of personal health. As we shall see in Chapter Three, public respect for the health professions has traditionally been substantial, as has been the public's willingness to trust professionals to make clinical decisions in the best interests of the patient. Historically, then, the health professions in the United States have enjoyed a munificent and stable environment shared by few, if any, other professions. Over the last two decades, however, several trends have been gathering strength, transforming this benign environment into one that is turbulent at best and hostile at worst.

Shifts in the Environment

Changes in the demographic, economic, cultural, governmental, and knowledge sectors of society are affecting the work of health professionals and fermenting concern about their role and contribution in the coming years.

Changing Economic Conditions

Economic conditions in the health industry have been altered by the seemingly unstoppable escalation of health care costs. As a percentage of GNP, health care expenditures rose an average of 0.14 per year for the time period 1950–1970, accelerating to 0.23 per year between 1970 and 1990. This escalation has dramatically affected federal, state, and local governments— whose health care expenditures in 1991 were 30.8 percent of total expenditures compared to 11.5 percent in 1965 (U.S. Department of Health and Human Services, 1993). Businesses spent 100.5 percent of corporate profits after taxes on health care in 1989 compared to 14 percent in 1965. Consumers were not unaffected, either, with health spending rising from 4.2 percent of adjusted personal income in 1965 to 5.1 percent in 1989 (Levit, Lazenby, Letsch, and Cowan, 1991). Moreover, between 31 and 36 million Americans had no health insurance on any given day in the late 1980s and even more were inadequately protected against the possibility of large medical bills (Friedman, 1991). No longer can health care professionals assume that businesses, government, and consumers will quietly agree to accept price increases without challenge.

The growing pool of dollars flowing into health care and the potential for large profits attracted big business to the health care industry in the 1970s. By 1986 private corporations owned 20 percent of the acute care hospitals and 67 percent of chronic care facilities (Wohl, 1989). In response to increasingly competitive conditions, hospitals have rapidly combined into vertically and horizontally integrated multiorganizational systems — a movement expected to encompass some 80 percent of the nation's hospitals by the year 2000 (Shortell, Morrison, and Friedman, 1990). Health professionals have thus been thrust into relationships with much larger and more powerful economic entities than the typical independent community hospital of the 1960s. For-profit entities, in particular, claim to create labor input efficiencies and management practices directed by business discipline (Frist and Howard, 1989), both of which may conflict with professionals' interests. In addition, groups of providers now have the size and economic incentive to invest in research on the cost-effectiveness of health professional services and use the results to shape practice.

Changing economic conditions have been another factor provoking major intervention by employers into the health care industry. Due to the impact of health care costs on corporate profits, corporations are attempting to manage health care utilization and costs through a variety of interventions, including contracting with providers to manage utilization and provide discounts, developing company health care facilities, lobbying legislatures, and encouraging competition among alternative providers (Hayes, 1989; Bergthold, 1990). Efforts to control costs have stimulated the growth of health maintenance organizations (HMOs), reflected in an enrollment growth from 9.1 million persons in 1980 to 33.6 million in 1990 (Kraus, Porter, and Ball, 1990); preferred provider organizations (PPOs) had become available as an option for some 60 million people by 1989; and other types of managed care, such as second opinion programs (ProPAC, 1990), began to appear.

Overall, the strains created by escalating health care costs have shifted the health care system from a condition of provider domination toward one of buyer domination (Light, 1991a, 1991b). Employers, government, and individual purchasers of health services are emphasizing cost containment and stricter scrutiny of quality of services at the expense of the professional pursuit of autonomy, income, and control over management and policy decisions.

Another outcome of climbing costs has been the encouragement of competition among providers of services, both organizations and individuals. Delivery organizations now have more incentive to substitute cheaper professionals for more expensive ones, and third-party reimbursers have the same incentives. As a result, the traditional division of labor, under the control of physicians and dentists, is crumbling. Indeed Blayney and Fitz (1990, p. 17) are prompted to conclude that "the assumption that all services of allied professions must be controlled by physicians is simply incorrect." Physical therapy is one allied health profession that has successfully challenged legal requirements that patients be seen only after a physician's referral or under a physician's supervision, and many allied health professions are moving toward independent practice (Hershey, 1987). Psychologists have achieved significant progress in their campaign to be granted the legal and fiscal privileges enjoyed by psychiatrists. Chapter Four discusses many other examples of this trend. Further evidence of increased competition is the extensive advertising now common in many local markets by health professionals of all types.

Rationalization of Knowledge

The rationalization of knowledge in many work domains has enabled greater bureaucratic control of credentialed experts and professionals in general (Murphy, 1990), and health professionals are no exception. Formal rationalization of knowledge emphasizes reliance on externally imposed rules, regulations, and laws — rather than professional norms and values — to create standardization in the application of knowledge and hence greater external control over it (Ritzer and Walczak, 1988).

Rationalization enables employers to intervene in the professional's task domains and even to educate their own work force or substitute nonhuman for human technology. Microelectronics and computers are providing management with a technology for standardizing and controlling professional work. More clinical professionals are finding themselves under the authority of managers trained in management schools rather than fellow professionals. Protocols for care and guidelines for clinical practice are becoming common, as government and health care organizations attempt to standardize care so that its quality and cost can be controlled or at least predicted with more accuracy (Field and Lohr, 1992; Longest, 1991).

In addition, employers are training their own workers in order to meet their particular needs. Humana, the large multihospital corporation, for example, has opened schools for licensed practical nurses ("Humana . . . ," 1990), and Beverly Enterprises, owner of some 880 nursing homes nationally, has training programs for nurse aides with a goal of providing some forty thousand new employees in a little more than two years ("Beverly . . . ," 1990). These and other large employers could introduce similar programs for other health professions.

The knowledge base of a profession is a public good accessible to interested consumers. The self-care movement encourages consumers to apply knowledge without the intervention of a professional. Consumers also are demanding a greater role in choosing among different health care providers. These trends pose a special challenge to professions that provide low-technology services, such as mental health counseling. The rise of the self-help movement in mental health reduces the quantity of potential buyers for the services of such professions as psychiatry, psychology, and medical social work. A similar challenge is presented to those professions whose knowledge base is easier to rationalize or whose services can be routinized. Optometry and ophthalmology, for example, are challenged by the consumer's new ability to buy off-the-shelf eyeglasses in retail drugstores.

To the extent that research dollars are devoted to prevention rather than cure of disease (a small but growing trend), the possibility of preventive treatment disrupts the predictability of the future supply of buyers to many professions. Dentistry, for example, faces reduced demand from the pediatric population due to the success of fluoride treatment and new dental sealant techniques. These technological developments shift the demand in the older adult population as well — away from crowns, bridges, and dentures toward fillings.

Two related developments in knowledge and technology

are affecting the health professions. Certainly the *speed* with which new knowledge and technologies are developing creates new uncertainties. Along with changes in knowledge and technology come potential revisions in the relative effectiveness of—and even the need for—a profession's services. The possibility of a professional's knowledge base becoming obsolete over his or her work life increases with the speed of change. In surgery, for example, the spread of lithotripsy, which permits management of many kidney stones without surgery, may reduce the number of surgeons required to be skilled in performing nephrolithotomies (Nash, 1987). An example of a broader change affects the profession of pharmacy, which finds reduced demand for traditional skills in mixing and dispensing drugs due to improvements in the technology of drug production and dispensing.

The other key development in the knowledge sector is the rise of expensive technologies. In professions reliant on expensive, high-tech devices, professionals sacrifice power to the suppliers of technology. Technological developments have made some health professionals dependent on expensive and complicated machines, such as sophisticated blood analyzers in medical laboratory technology, that they can neither afford to purchase nor keep operational themselves. Hence they must depend on large-scale institutions to purchase the equipment and depend on suppliers to maintain it and even train professionals in its use.

Changing Social Values

In general, the late 1970s and the 1980s saw a revival of free-market ideology in American society, as reflected in President Reagan's deregulation and privatization rhetoric and policy actions such as the deregulation of the airline and telephone industries. Even as the extremes of this philosophy have been rejected in the 1990s, the acceptance of "regulated competition" as preferable to "regulation" is widespread. Consumers and politicians are more likely to view monopolies and cartels as self-interested protectionism—and thus to challenge their continuance. This shift in values has helped propel the health care industry into a more competitive mode. A growing body of anti-elitist and anti-professional literature (for example, Illich, 1976; Derber, Schwartz, and Magrass, 1990) argues that professionals usurp the consumer's personal responsibility and create an unhealthy dependence on the expert.

Consumers have become more critical, too, of the health professions' contribution to social welfare. In regard to physicians, Light (1991b, p. 60) characterizes the change as a shift from "sacred trust in doctors" to "distrust of doctors' values, decisions, even competence." Starr (1982, p. 380), tracing the origins of this trend to the 1970s, points to a "diminished faith in the efficacy of medicine and increased concern about its relation to other moral values." There is little doubt that this trend has continued since the 1970s. For instance, national survey data report high consumer dissatisfaction with the role of health professionals in controlling costs and creating access to care ("Opinion . . . ," 1991).

The change in society's values is reflected in the language of new health professional licensing laws being implemented in the Province of Ontario, Canada. Ministry of Health publications argue that the new system "is based on the principle that the sole purpose of regulation is to protect the public interest, and not to enhance any profession's economic power or raise its status. The existing system . . . does not effectively protect the public" (Ministry of Health, Ontario, 1989, p. 3). The ministry even claims that the new system will lead to "the elimination of status distinctions among health professions" (Ministry of Health, Ontario, 1991). These changes are being studied by several state governments in the United States.

More Invasive Government Policy

Revisions in the Ontario licensing laws are an example of a final category of challenges to the health professions — more invasive policies of government toward the health professions. While supplying new resources to the health professions, federal legislation such as the Health Professions Educational Assistance Act of 1963 served notice that professions were not meeting society's goals for access to services. At the federal level, government policy began a slow shift from support of the health professions to control with the 1971 Comprehensive Health Manpower Training Act (Lostetter and Chapman, 1979). Rather than providing lump sums to health professional schools, the law provided that schools would receive a fixed sum of money for each student in return for agreeing to boost the school's enrollment by a fixed percentage. Schools of medicine, osteopathy, dentistry, veterinary medicine, optometry, pharmacy, and podiatry were covered. Even more directive in terms of shaping the flow of entrants into the health professions was the 1976 Health Professions Educational Assistance Act, which required the nation's medical schools to have 50 percent of their graduates entering primary care residencies by 1980.

Federal backing for the development of physician assistants and nurse practitioners in the 1970s was further evidence of government's desire to induce more accessible services. Professional standards review organizations, established in 1972 to monitor the quality of care rendered to recipients of federal health programs, were an early foray into the traditional territory of the health professions as well. Federal intervention in monitoring the quality of health professionals continued with authorization of a National Practitioner Data Bank in 1986. The data bank, which began in earnest in 1990, collects records of adverse actions against physicians, dentists, and other professionals relating to malpractice payments, licensure, and clinical privileges (Anthony and Crowley, 1991).

The Medicare Prospective Payment System (PPS) legislation implemented after 1983 has directly or indirectly affected most health professionals. The PPS legislation fixed levels of hospital reimbursement for 468 diagnosis-related groups of conditions, giving hospitals sudden incentives to minimize a patient's length of stay and the resources dispensed. Practitioners whose skills could hasten a patient's exit from the hospital (such as respiratory therapists) and administrative personnel (such as medical record administrators) gained in relative importance to the hospital's profitability. Moreover, this legislation gave hospitals greater incentives to substitute cheaper providers for more expensive ones. Federal control of reimbursement was expanded in 1989 when, as part of its Medicare reforms, Congress created new volume performance standards to control total outlays to physicians and began the process of creating a new Medicare resource-based relative value fee schedule that is based more on the actual costs of care than on prevailing charges. Federal government influence over the reimbursement and delivery system no doubt will continue to expand, as the Clinton administration and legislators seek new ways to increase access and control costs.

With respect to new knowledge, the federal Agency for Health Care Policy and Research is responsible for the development of practice guidelines for several health professions' treatment of costly illnesses. The National Institutes of Health consensus development process has similar aims. With only 10 to 20 percent of health care procedures documented to be beneficial by controlled clinical trials, the possibilities for research and intervention into practice patterns are monumental (Hillman, 1987).

Both the Federal Trade Commission (FTC) and the Justice Department have acted to curb anticompetitive activities by suing hospitals, medical societies, physicians, and dentists for antitrust infractions. The medical staff of a Savannah, Georgia, hospital was challenged for denying a nurse-midwife's hospital privileges, for example, and two MD allergists in Texas were challenged for organizing a boycott against drug manufacturers that were marketing new allergy products to nonallergists ("Another Force . . . ," 1991). The FTC has hammered away at state advertising restrictions and commercial practice restrictions since the 1970s, particularly in the dental and vision care markets. The FTC also continues to urge state governments to view with skepticism the claims of professions seeking or maintaining self-regulation through licensure: "Even the situations in which licensing increases the quality of the licensee-provided service, consumers are not necessarily better off," the FTC notes, because of price increases that are related to the quality improvements (Cox and Foster, 1990, p. viii).

A more invasive policy is reflected not only in the federal government but in the judiciary and in state government as well. In the courts, new interpretations of government policy countenance a more competitive marketplace for the health professions. The courts began to encourage competition within and among professions in the 1970s by such decisions as *Goldfarb* v. *Virginia State Bar* (1975), invalidating minimum fee schedules used by bar associations, *Bates* v. *State Bar of Arizona* (1977), striking down advertising restrictions against lawyers, and *Virginia State Board of Pharmacy* v. *Virginia Citizens Consumer Council* (1976), allowing drug price advertising. In 1987, after a long court battle, the American Medical Association, American College of Radiologists, and American College of Surgeons were found guilty of antitrust and conspiracy in their efforts to restrain the practice of chiropractic medicine.

Federal efforts to persuade states to limit licensing of new health professions began in the 1970s (U.S. Department of Health, Education, and Welfare, 1971, 1977a), and states began to perform sunset reviews of licensing boards, add public members to boards, and exert more administrative scrutiny over licensing boards (Carpenter, 1987). As well, public concern has prompted many of the professions to develop continuing education or recertification or relicensure requirements. A more extensive reform of state licensing systems, under study in several states, would be based on the Ontario reforms mentioned earlier. Such a system would license only the potentially harmful acts performed by health professionals, rather than the whole work domain traditionally claimed by the profession. The Province of Ontario has compiled a list of such harmful acts, as well as the different professions that will be allowed to perform them. As a result, for instance, both midwives and physicians are permitted to perform uncomplicated deliveries; both audiologists and physicians can prescribe hearing aids; both dentists and denturists can dispense dentures. All acts that are not on the "potentially hazardous" list can be performed by anyone (Ministry of Health, Ontario, 1991).

Demographic Shifts

A final source of environmental change is the shifting demographic composition of the population. Two key developments are the increasing proportion of the population that is elderly and the increasing racial and ethnic diversity of the population.

The percentage of the population aged sixty-five and over rose from 8 percent to 12.3 percent between 1950 and 1990 and is expected to grow to 20.1 percent by the year 2030 (Congressional Budget Office, 1992). This development shifts the needs and demands of patients to such areas as rehabilitation therapy, home care, and long-term care.

By the year 2000, some 30 percent of Americans are expected to be members of a racial minority (Shugars, O'Neil, and Bader, 1991). During the 1980–1988 period, the Asian-American, Hispanic-American, Native American, and African-American populations each increased at more than double the rate of the white population (National Center for Health Statistics, 1991). Racial and ethnic diversity creates new demands for treatment of health problems that are particularly acute in certain populations, such as the problem of hypertension in African-Americans, and calls for practitioners who belong to the different ethnic or racial groups. A related movement is the demand for health care services designed directly for women's particular needs and provided by professionals more sensitive to these needs than has been the case.

A further challenge to the health professions arises from the changing health characteristics of the population. The higher prevalence of chronic conditions faced by the elderly population, such as arthritis and Alzheimer's disease, and the growing numbers of AIDS patients, are examples of the changing needs of the population that require response from the health professions.

New Relationships with Key Stakeholders

New developments in different sectors of the environment have altered the work setting of health professionals in fundamental ways. The general environmental changes discussed so far can be summarized as follows:

Economic Conditions

- Escalation of health care costs
- Greater provider competition
- Business and insurer efforts to control costs

Knowledge and Technology

- Rationalization of knowledge
- Employer sponsorship of educational programs
- Increased consumer access to knowledge; more self-care
- Discoveries of preventive methods
- Increased speed of new knowledge development
- Proliferation of expensive technologies

Social Values

- Monopolies and cartels viewed with suspicion
- Distrust of professionals

Government Policy

- Modify numbers and specialties of health professionals; improve access
- Constrain growth of Medicare and Medicaid costs
- Develop practice guidelines
- Encourage competition among professionals
- Discourage licensing

Demography

- Increasing racial and ethnic diversity
- Aging of the population
- New disease patterns

The diversity and breadth of these changes make them difficult to assess systematically in relation to the strategic adaptation of professions. One way to organize these new developments is to trace their impact on the key relationships in which professions are engaged. To do so, we use the concept of the *stakeholder* — an individual, group, or organization that has a stake in the decisions and actions of an organization and may attempt to influence them (Blair and Fottler, 1990, p. 4). Stakeholders can be inside an organization (the employees, for instance), external to it, or both inside and outside — that is, at the interface between an organization and its environment. Changes in the general environment are played out in relationships between stakeholders and organizations.

A similar concept is the *task environment*. The task environment has been defined apropos to organizations as "those aspects of the general environment relevant to the organization's goal setting and goal attainment. It can be defined specifically in terms of its customers, suppliers, employees, competitors, and government regulatory agencies" (Bedeian and Zammuto, 1991, p. 318).

Adapting the concept of stakeholder to apply to professions, we argue that professionals and their associations interact with five key external and interface stakeholders: substitutes, suppliers of equipment and products, suppliers of knowledge (teachers and researchers), buyers, and regulators. The relationships are depicted in Figure 1.1. In this section, we describe these major groups of stakeholders and indicate ways in which a profession's changing relationships with these stakeholders reflect the general trends described earlier.

Figure 1.1. Key External and Interface Stakeholders.

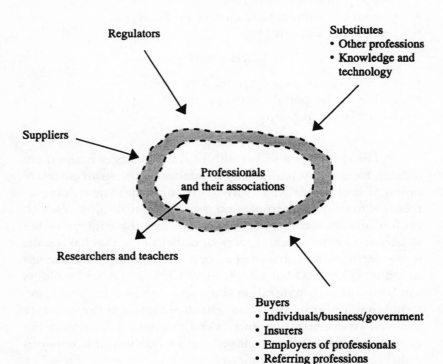

Substitutes

Substitutes are the alternative ways in which consumers can meet the purposes served by the professional. In some work domains, substitute professions compete for the same buyers. Optometrists and ophthalmologists, orthopedic surgeons and chiropractors and physical therapists, and psychologists and psychiatrists are examples of professions that are substitutes in some areas of service. Other substitutes may not be professionals, however. If consumers can achieve improvement in dental health by greater use of fluoride or dental sealants or flossing, these products and services and their vendors become substitutes for the services of dentists. Self-care is a substitute for many of the low-technology services of professionals, such as diet counseling.

Of the five key external stakeholders, the relationship with substitutes traditionally has received the most attention from health professions, particularly in their early years. In the past, much of a profession's early activity was directed at building barriers to protect it from the threats of other professional substitutes. Professions typically have achieved this by defining areas of jurisdiction in which other professions are not allowed to foray (Abbott, 1988).

Now, however, the importance of the challenges from substitutes must be weighed in the context of the far more complex environment described earlier. The creation of substitutes for professions has powerful support from external stakeholders, initiated by the relentless upswing in the price of services and the ideological shift toward competition. Buyers and regulators now press for competition between professions and substitutes as a means of controlling costs and increasing access. Therefore, professions are being thrown into substitute relationships more than ever before — and they must deal with these relationships differently than they have in the past. In particular, medicine's declining dominance of the health division of labor contributes to more competition from substitutes. One observer, Birenbaum (1990, p. 4), claims that "a new division of labor is emerging in which physicians may have to share responsibility for health-care with the new practitioners [for example, nurse practitioners and physician assistants] rather than simply delegating tasks."

Suppliers

Suppliers provide the resources that are inputs to the professional's work. These include such organizations as laboratories, equipment manufacturers, and the makers and distributors of products like visionwear and pharmaceuticals that are in turn processed and dispensed by health practitioners. In general, the strategic challenge presented by suppliers has been negligible for most of the health professions, as suppliers rarely have ventured downstream into the delivery of services. But in cases where suppliers can offer services directly to buyers and bypass the professional, as has occurred particularly in pharmacy, the profession faces critical challenges.

Teachers and Researchers

The concept of suppliers also can be conceptualized at the level of the profession as a whole. The suppliers of *knowledge* to the profession are its teachers and researchers. As we shall see in Chapters Two and Seven, most health professions have been successful in integrating the teachers and researchers into the profession, and creating shared goals with them. To the extent that teachers, researchers, and their organizations are integrated into the profession, it can more easily maintain control over its size, the content of educational curricula and practice, and educational socialization into its norms. But such control can be exerted to the detriment of the profession if society's needs — for changing curricula and more practitioners, for example — are ignored. The recent development of research entities largely outside the professions, as well as the growing interest of buyers, regulators, and employers in the training of professionals, requires new attention to the suppliers of knowledge.

Buyers

Buyers are those who pay for the services of health professionals: the organizations that employ professionals, the patients who directly purchase services, and the third parties that reimburse patients or professionals. To the extent that buyers are available only on referral from other professionals, referring professionals are indirect buyers of services too.

For many health professions, perhaps the most significant pressure in the long term will come from the buyers of services. As noted earlier, this pressure is tied to a combination of factors: the growing size and complexity of many buyers (especially hospitals); the magnified emphasis on cost containment that strengthens the position of those who are in an administrative position to manipulate the levers of bureaucratic control; and the explosion of costly technology, the power over which is increasingly being transferred to the buyer side. Employers are gaining more power to intervene in the work domain of professionals — a shift that has been deemed "the central development of modern work history" (Abbott, 1988, p. 275). Organized groups of buyers and insurers, as well as individuals, are questioning the relative emphasis on treatment rather than prevention and health promotion in such areas as health research and reimbursement of services. As noted earlier, growing numbers of people without health insurance, as well as members of racial and ethnic minorities and persons with chronic conditions, are seeking care — posing further challenges in the relationship between buyers and health professionals.

Besides, in contrast to the limited likelihood of downstream integration suggested in the case for suppliers, there is a real possibility of upstream integration stemming from the buyer side. This is taking different forms, many of which are being summarized under the title of "managed care." Hospitals, the primary buyer of the services of many health professionals, are key stakeholders in the formation or control of the growing numbers of health maintenance organizations, preferred provider organizations, and other forms of managed care systems. The power of hospitals in this area is further reinforced by the significant role being played by their buyers: the health insurance companies. Hospitals and other delivery organizations are in a position to shift the balance of power and clinical roles among the members of certain professions and their possible substitutes.

Regulators

Professions operate within a social and economic system regulated by the state. Regulatory organizations monitor entry into the professions and the quality of practice. In the United States, significant regulation occurs at the state as well as the federal level. State licensing boards, and ultimately state legislatures, have formal authority over much of the work of professionals. The judiciary too is a state-sanctioned form of regulatory control over the professions. Some voluntary agencies are developed without formal state authority, although they generally achieve different levels of formal recognition. The JCAHO, for example, is a voluntary accreditation organization for hospitals whose survey results are used by many state and federal agencies to judge qualification for government programs (Affeldt, 1980).

Historically, the health professions have been quite successful at achieving agreements with the state that delegate regulatory powers to the professions themselves. Achieving self-regulation is an important step in the process of attaining legitimacy, a process covered in Chapter Three. Like other external stakeholders, however, regulators are presenting new challenges to the health professions, including challenges to self-regulation. Studies of the effects of licensing laws generally have demonstrated that many licensing regulations benefit the interests of practitioners rather than consumers (Gaumer, 1984; Begun and Feldman, 1990). Revisions to state licensing systems, described earlier, are an example of the more equivocal relationships now unfolding between regulators and health professions. Other indicators are the increasingly common presence of significant numbers of lay members of licensing and regulatory boards, as well as the centralization of administrative control over licensing at the state level.

Implications of Changing Conditions

Benign environmental conditions—the expansion of a client base, the explosion of specialized knowledge and technology, abundant financing, public respect and trust, and formal government support and protection — created a secure work world for the health professions from their inception through the 1960s. This shield of benevolence insulated them from major disruption and buffered them from external pressures. At the individual level, health care professionals were effectively sheltered from economic competition from their peers or substitutes. Relationships with stakeholders generally were stable and supportive.

Changing conditions have considerably altered this picture. As reviewed in the preceding pages, professionals are losing their traditional control of certain relationships — with members of their own profession and members of substitute professions who increasingly compete for the same customers; with the more powerful and businesslike hospitals and multiorganizational health systems in which they work, as the organizations seek to rationalize and control their production processes; with suppliers of knowledge and technology; with government regulators who seek greater availability and cost-effectiveness in the delivery of professional services; and with the buyers of their services who openly challenge their judgments about prices, quality, and efficacy.

Equally important as a challenge to the health professions is the expanding interconnection or density of linkages among the stakeholders. Alliances between suppliers and employers of professionals, or between buyers and researchers, represent much stronger challenges to the health professions than do isolated pressures from each of the stakeholders alone. This trend increases the uncertainty faced by professions, since they can no longer manage simple one-to-one relationships with these stakeholders.

To attend to all these new demands and take advantage of new opportunities, new strategies are needed for managing relationships with stakeholders. To argue that professions should be concerned about "strategies" and "stakeholders" implies that professions function in some ways as organizations do. In the next chapter, a profession is conceptualized as a collective that has a structure and pursues strategies. The idea that a profession is a collective is an important step in mobilizing professionals and their associations toward new patterns of strategic adaptation.

Chapter Two ◆ ◆ ◆ ◆ ◆

Structure and Strategy in the Professional Community

Thus far, we have referred to health professions as though they were corporate entities engaging in relationships with external stakeholders and acting strategically. Before proceeding further, it is important to understand the nature of this corporate entity. After assessing the structure of professions, we elaborate on the concept of strategy as it applies to them. Together with the concepts of the general environment and key stakeholders introduced in Chapter One, these ideas form a framework for understanding strategic adaptation in the health professions.

Professions as Communities

As individuals, professionals pursue goals such as income, autonomy at work, prestige, or serving society. They share many of these goals with other professionals, of course, and aggregate into professional associations to advance these common goals. Individual members of professions use voting privileges, personal influence, or subgroup pressure politics to influence the direction of their associations and the profession as a whole. Within a single profession, separate associations may form to represent the distinctive goals of segments differentiated by specialty, professional setting (for example, hospital pharmacists versus community pharmacists), or other attributes such as minority racial status. In addition to associations comprised of practitioners, educators or researchers often form organizations relating to specific professions.

The individuals and associations in a profession are loosely coupled. It is this fragile aspect of professions that was emphasized by Bucher and Strauss (1961, p. 326) in their depiction of professions as "loose amalgamations of segments pursuing different objectives in different manners and more or less delicately held together under a common name at a particular period in history." Loose coupling means that elements of the community are linked but "are also subject to spontaneous changes and preserve some degree of independence and indeterminacy" (Orton and Weick, 1990, p. 204).

Coupling derives in part from the shared goals. But professionals are also bonded to each other by virtue of the similar education and training they receive and the type of work they do. In the words of Freidson (1986, pp. 210–211), this in fact distinguishes occupations from professions: "Most occupations can be characterized as a mere aggregate of practitioners or jobholders. . . . It is different for professions. First, they have an occupational community that extends beyond any particular workplace, a community sustained by a common credential, common interest in preserving shared privileges, common specialized training and shared occupation identity, and the like." Others have noted the "conscious parallelism" created among professionals by their geographic proximity in local markets and common educational, social, and professional activities (Evans, 1980).

In order to emphasize the shared, cooperative, and interdependent nature of the elements of a profession, we will use the term professional community interchangeably with the term profession. A *professional community* is the loosely coupled network of individual professionals pursuing shared goals and their associations. The notion of a professional community pushes the meaning of profession beyond a mere aggregate of individual practitioners and emphasizes its corporate character (Freidson,

1989, p. 190). Such a conceptualization is important for strategic adaptation, because it encourages professionals to treat their profession as a strategic entity. If we can apply to health professional communities the basic concepts and tools of strategic analysis that are applied to organizations, we may well discover strategic approaches that will help them adapt to change.

Boundaries

The core of the professional community is the full-time practitioners and their professional associations. The professional community may also encompass certain individuals and associations at the fringes of the community, however, such as regulators, employers, administrators, educators, and researchers. Stakeholders in these positions may relate to the profession as external entities, or they may be incorporated to varying degrees into the community. To some extent, the professions incorporate into the community many of the people and organizations that regulate them (peer review organizations, accrediting bodies, licensing boards), conduct education and research, and administer their work (for example, clinician department heads and MD–CEOs in hospitals).

     In this book, regulators are considered external stakeholders because of their ultimate accountability to the state, which is a force outside the profession. Employers and administrators are regarded as external "buyers" of the professional's services, but since many professionals are employed by organizations owned or administered by themselves or their peers, employers or administrators may be incorporated to some extent in the professional community. Educators and researchers more commonly are integrated into the professional community of practitioners, and they are considered to be both internal and external to the professional community, depending on the profession. As roles shift, the degree to which these fringe elements are integrated into the professional community, as well as boundaries of the community, may change. But the core of the community — its practitioners and their associations — remains.

Subcommunities

The differentiation of the professional community by specialty, work setting, and geography raises important questions for the analysis of strategies. We refer to these differentiated segments as subcommunities. As strategies and management practices may vary across subcommunities, it is not easy to characterize an overall professional community. Specialties within nursing, for example, have their own professional associations with their own strategies, and practitioners may pursue strategies that relate more to their specialty than to the profession as a whole. Within a profession, segments may compete or collaborate depending on the strategic issue they face. Both commercial and professional optometrists (segments within the profession of optometry) compete in some markets for the same customers, for example, but they face similar substitute threats from ophthalmologists (MDs). Members of such segments can overlook internal differences if an external threat is serious.

Adding to the complexity, different strategic issues involve different segments within professions. The issue of reimbursement for vision care, for example, strategically affects ophthalmology, a medical specialty, much more than other specialties within medicine. But this is little different than the position of national or international business firms, which have national or regional or product line divisions with strategies and management practices of their own that must be coordinated with the larger corporation's overall ("corporate") strategy and structure. In this book our focus is on the professional community itself rather than its various subcommunities. To the extent that subcommunities are independent of the focal community, however, many of the issues we discuss are germane to them.

Subcommunities may or may not be considered separate professions. Medical social work could be defined as a subcommunity within the larger community of social work, for example, or as a community of its own. Nurse-midwifery may be a community of its own; it could also be considered a subcommunity within nursing. For our purposes, the judgment about when one community ends and another begins is based on the degree to which distinctive internal structures and external relationships can be differentiated. For example, we consider the internal structure and the external relationships of long-term-care administrators to be sufficiently different from those of health care administrators to define them as a separate profession.

Professionals may very well belong to more than one professional community or subcommunity. Medical specialists, for example, often identify with their specialty association more than the primary association. Further, the relationship between subcommunities and communities may change. Subcommunities may split off and form separate professional communities, as dispensing opticians split from opticianry and evolved into optometry. At other times, separate communities may unite, as osteopathy and allopathic medicine (MDs) have attempted, with the smaller partner becoming a new subcommunity within the larger community.

Professional communities and subcommunities can be examined at any level of aggregation—local, state, regional, national, or international. Although few professions are tightly coupled across national boundaries, this situation is changing and we can expect the further development of global professional communities in the future, a trend discussed in Chapter Seven. Health care, like most retail products and services, is delivered primarily within local markets. It is in the local community that patients visit the various organizations and professionals involved in health care, where referral networks are based, and where competition occurs (Luke, 1992; Luke and Begun, 1987; Seidel, Seavey, and Lewis, 1989). At the state level, most health professions form organizational units and engage in important relationships with regulators and buyer groups.

But it is at the national level that the conceptualization of health professions as communities is most germane. At the national level, health professionals and their associations stand as a collective of otherwise highly fragmented workers to adapt to the new challenges and opportunities described in Chapter One. In this book, as we focus primarily on the professional communities themselves, we concentrate on strategy and structure at the national level. We have described the profession as a loosely coupled community. To further investigate the nature of professional communities, we next identify the important dimensions of their internal structure.

Internal Structure

Scott (1992, pp. 16–17) says that all collectivities have both normative and behavioral *structures* that link participants in patterned activities, interactions, and sentiments. Structures form the framework for collective activity. In this sense, the structure of a profession includes both its differentiation into segments and those elements that integrate the differentiated parts—for instance, its culture, organization, goals, and knowledge base. Other important features of professions that affect their patterned activities are their size and the common personal traits of members, such as race and gender, which we also consider to be structural attributes. Here we list the key internal characteristics of professions:

- Size
- Distribution of personal attributes (gender, race, and so on)
- Vertical differentiation (by position, experience, educational level, and so on)
- Horizontal differentiation (by geography, specialty, practice setting and so on)
- Knowledge base
- Culture
- Organization of individuals into associations
- Organizational field of associations
- Collective goals

The internal structure of a profession places important constraints on its ability to adapt strategically. Unorganized professions are at a disadvantage in conflicts with organized professions. Female-dominated professions have faced greater obstacles than male-dominated ones. At the same time, internal structural characteristics can serve as the foundation for strategic

initiatives. The internal "parts" of the profession become some
of its major tools. Manipulation of the profession's size, knowledge base, and culture, for example, is often the key to responding to new environmental demands. Moreover, professions strive
to create harmony and cohesion in order to pursue collective
activity. As a first step, professional communities must understand their internal dimensions and their effect on the fit between the professional community and its environment.

Size

A key structural variable is the size of the professional community, roughly indicated by the number of individual professionals. The size of health professions varies widely, as was
shown in Table 1.1 in Chapter One. Registered nursing is by far
the largest U.S. health profession, followed by medicine (MDs).
Radiologic technologists, medical technologists, pharmacists,
and dentists comprise fairly large professions, as well, each with
more than 100,000 members. By contrast, the professions of
medical record administration, nurse-midwifery, podiatry, and
physician assisting are small in numbers, with 20,000 or fewer
members.

The size of a professional community has numerous implications for its other structural attributes and its strategies.
As size increases, the profession is harder to control as a strategic entity. Integration is threatened simply by the difficulty
of communication and coordination within the profession. More
resources must be expended in order to create a collective value
structure and to participate in collective action. Besides, as additional members differ from present members in age, back-
ground, and employment setting, the possibility of conflicting
goals within the profession grows and individual members are
less likely to agree on professional norms and strategies.

Size changes the relationships with external stakeholders
as well. As size increases, members of the profession are more
likely to encounter substitute professionals in their local markets. If size exceeds demand by too great a gap, professionals
may lose power relative to buyers. But some minimal size is

necessary if a profession is to establish power in its relationships with external stakeholders. In both local and national markets, size is a key source of power in relationships with suppliers and buyers. Greater size enables a profession to respond to demands from buyers for accessibility. Greater size allows a professional community to argue that it represents a significant portion of a buyer's market — the argument that optometrists are accessible to a large portion of the primary vision care market, for instance, helped optometry to achieve recognition for Medicare reimbursement by the federal government. Greater size provides a basis for collective organization at all levels — professions with few practitioners in local communities, for example, are less able to develop strong local professional associations that can influence state and federal representatives and other important stakeholders. Greater size facilitates the spreading of one's message to the general public, to specific groups of potential buyers, and to political elites. And, finally, greater size allows for the accumulation of enough resources to hire specialists to provide strategic direction to the profession. Otherwise, designing strategy is a part-time or voluntary activity of selected practitioners.

Distribution of Personal Attributes

Another dimension of professions that has implications for strategic adaptation is the collective personal characteristics of individual members, such as their gender and race. Professions face pressures to accept all interested and qualified candidates regardless of gender, race, and the like. Yet in the United States, as is the case with business organizations, professional communities with large proportions of white males have been the most successful. No powerful health professions have high proportions of females or racial minorities. The failure of several health professions to fully achieve professional status has been attributed by some observers to the fact that they are predominantly female and thus elicit opposition from powerful male elites (Ritzer, 1977). In fact, one might argue that the goals of professionalization itself are a construction of male in-groups and are not necessarily shared by professions that are predominantly female or out-group dominated (Abbott and Wallace, 1990; Lorentzon, 1990; Witz, 1992). The distribution of attributes such as gender shapes the profession's response to environmental demands.

Vertical Differentiation

Another key dimension of internal structure is differentiation within the professional community, a topic we introduced earlier in this chapter by noting the existence of subcommunities. The extent of differentiation within a community has important implications.

The divisions within the professional community generally move in two directions — vertically and horizontally. First, we consider vertical differentiation. Segments within a profession may differ according to their authority over other segments of the profession. Such divisions are based on members' formal position or the degree of their education, training, or experience. Nursing, defined broadly, is the most vertically differentiated of the health professions — ranging from the most educated teachers and practitioners (doctoral degree) to advanced-level practitioners (master's degree) to registered nurses (bachelor's degree or diploma or associate degree) to licensed practical nurses (generally one year of post–high school education) to the least educated nurse aides and assistants.

Vertical differentiation creates different interests relative to external stakeholders. The academic segment of a profession, for example, often is more isolated from the market forces impinging on practitioners. Or those at the bottom of the vertical hierarchy are more likely to oppose raising entry standards, as licensed practical nurses have done within nursing. Internal cohesion in medicine is threatened by the vertical differentiation introduced by physician administrators of quality assurance controls. Physician administrators may be assigned formal hierarchical authority over the clinical work of other physicians, and physician administrators may have interests close to those of the buyers of physician services and the employers of physicians (Freidson, 1985).

Sooner or later, most professions face critical decisions

about vertical differentiation, such as whether technical-level personnel should be created inside or outside the professional community. Pharmacy technicians are primarily being educated outside the formal pharmacy education system, for instance, via on-the-job training (Sorkin, 1989). The profession of pharmacy wrestles with the question of whether to bring them into its fold or not. Another common dilemma involves the differentiation potentially introduced by the raising of entry standards: should experienced practitioners be excused ("grandfathered" in) when entry standards are raised? The outcomes of these decisions become constraints on further changes in the profession's strategies and structures.

While vertical differentiation opens the door to increased internal conflict, it may be undertaken purposely in order to satisfy internal or external stakeholder demands. The creation of doctorally prepared teachers within the profession responds to practitioners' demands to be taught by members of their own community, for example, and it facilitates the profession's ability to integrate new knowledge and technology.

Horizontal Differentiation

Also important are horizontal divisions in professions, usually based on specialty, type of employer, geography, or practice setting. Pharmacists, for example, are represented by separate professional associations for hospital pharmacists and for community pharmacists, as well as an all-encompassing professional association. Chiropractors have traditionally been segmented into "mixed" and "straight" groups, each with its own professional organization. Most large professions have numerous specialty divisions: medicine, for example, has twenty-three such divisions with their own specialty certification board, such as plastic surgery, urology, and family practice.

Such divisions provide the basis for potential conflicts of interest relative to new entrants, buyers, suppliers, and substitutes. For example, the differing interests of primary care physicians and surgeons regarding the federal government's Resource-Based Relative Value Fee Schedule (RBRVS) for Medicare created internal strife regarding medicine's strategic response to the RBRVS proposal. Public health physicians are differentiated from other physicians by virtue of preventive medicine specialization and their salaried employment by government agencies, and their organizations often adopt strategic positions antithetical to those of other physicians. Similarly, commercial and professional segments within optometry differed on the profession's response to the FTC's attempts to stimulate market competition within the profession and between optometry and other vision care providers.

Another source of horizontal differentiation is the geographic dispersion of members. Geographic dispersion affects the profession's ability to communicate and coordinate and places stress on internal cohesion. But as with size, appropriate geographic dispersion can serve as a source of strength relative to stakeholders. Buyers' demands for service often include a geographic component, for instance. Many buyers of health care services, particularly governments, demand wide dispersion of health care professionals since health care is a basic need of all individuals. Geographic dispersion across political jurisdictions can be an advantage in political fights. The large number of nurses, and their geographic dispersion, enable the nursing profession to organize effectively at the grass-roots level. Using a military analogy, members of a profession must be allocated to local garrisons in order to establish power bases on new frontiers. The geographic dispersion of members over political and economic battle grounds is relevant to a profession's ability to engage substitutes, buyers, and sellers dispersed across those areas. To the extent that strategies are implemented at local or state levels, professional community members must be dispersed across those jurisdictions. The need for extensive geographic dispersion is apparent in many health professions as they increasingly face local challenges from buyers and substitutes.

Knowledge Base

Characteristics of the knowledge base are usually the foundation for distinguishing professions from occupations. Professions base their claim to special status on their possession of problem-solving knowledge, whether that claim is real or symbolic (Torstendahl, 1990). Professions have been defined as "exclusive occupational groups applying somewhat abstract knowledge to particular cases" (Abbott, 1988, p. 8). To demarcate the boundaries of our framework, in this book we define professions as occupations for which higher education about a specific work domain is a prerequisite to employment in particular positions. (For similar definitions, see Freidson, 1986, p. 59, and Hofoss, 1986, p. 202.) Higher education, as a source of legitimated and specialized knowledge, gives professionals the ability to claim autonomy in a specific work domain, as they can claim to possess knowledge about that work that nonprofessionals do not have.

The existence of higher education as a *prerequisite* to employment implies that the occupation exerts control over entry. In fact, it is useful to conceive of professions as occupations that have successfully pursued a strategy of professionalizing—that is, insisting on higher education about specific tasks as a prerequisite to employment in certain positions. Professions, then, differ from other occupations only in their choice of a strategy (professionalizing) and their success in attaining it. The successful profession achieves a labor market shelter, a social closure, or a sinecure for the occupation's members in the labor market (Freidson, 1986, p. 59). All of the health professions listed earlier in Table 1.1 have college-level educational programs, of at least two years in length, as the most common pathway to entry. While educational credentials are not always formally required for employment of the professionals listed in Table 1.1, in those cases possession of the higher education credentials does significantly improve chances for employment and frequently is a de facto prerequisite. In health care administration, for example, most current hospital administrators hold the master's degree, even though there is no legal requirement for it.

Professions differ from other occupations in their strategic adaptation because their structure and strategy are influenced by the need to maintain a distinctive and abstract knowledge base that is accessible only through higher education and is a prerequisite for employment. As a result, many of the strategies we discuss in this book deal with the development and control of knowledge. The knowledge bases of the many health professions differ in important ways. Above all, they differ in the degree to which they are subject to routinization. As we shall see in later chapters, professions are threatened when their knowledge base becomes routinized, as it opens them to challenge from substitutes — either in the form of machines or lower-priced workers — and to challenge from buyers or suppliers. Family nurse practitioners can perform the routine work of physicians, for example. Optometrists and ophthalmologists face a challenge from automatic refracting machines and from the consumer's ability to select eyeglasses by trial and error from store displays. Health care administrators, on the other hand, perform work that is quite varied and difficult to routinize, making this a less critical issue for the profession.

But if a knowledge base is too uncertain and too difficult to routinize, it is subject to the objection that it cannot be efficaciously applied. Psychiatry, for instance, faces this criticism in its counseling tasks. A useful way to classify the routinization of a profession's knowledge base is the indetermination/technicality (I/T) ratio proposed by Jamous and Peloille (1970). Technicality refers to the part played in the production process by means that can be measured and communicated in the form of rules; indetermination refers to the part played by means that escape rules. In dealing strategically with external stakeholders, an optimal level of the I/T ratio would be moderate, or moderate-high, rather than high. (See also Abbott, 1988, pp. 98–111.)

A related characteristic of professions is their dependence on machinery in the process of applying their knowledge base. Dependence on machines, as we shall see in Chapter Five, opens a profession to the possibility of vertical integration by suppliers.

Culture

Another important internal feature of a professional community is its culture — the shared norms, values, beliefs, and assumptions of its members. As Chapter Seven points out, culture is a key instrument for creating integration and a key tool in the strategic adaptation process. The negative effects of internal differentiation can be overcome if individuals and associations in the community share norms of cooperation. A strong internal culture of cooperation and collective mission can overcome differentiation and allow the professional community to present a united front in managing external demands. For example, many of the health professions have cultivated an underdog image in relation to medicine; chiropractic has used the image to galvanize internal strength. Even highly segmented professions can come together around a common challenge if they have a strong shared culture. The united opposition of nursing to the American Medical Association's proposal to create a new occupation, registered care technicians, is a good example of that process.

Organization

The professional communities of health professionals are variously organized. In some communities, most practitioners are involved in their primary professional association. In others, the primary association receives little support from individuals and there are diverse professional associations pursuing divergent agendas. In such settings, decisions about the community's strategy and structure emerge in a manner similar to the "social choice" context for decision making described by Warren (1967, pp. 403–404):

> [The social choice context] is exemplified by the autonomous behavior of a number of organizations and individuals in the community as they relate themselves and their behavior to any particular issue which concerns more than one of them. . . . There is no formal inclusive structure within which the units make their decisions; rather, decisions are made at the level of the units themselves, many of which may be inclusive organizations of a unitary, federative, or coalitional type. . . . There is no for-

mally structured provision for division of labor
within an inclusive context, each unit pursuing its
own goals and organizing itself for that purpose as
it deems appropriate.

Because the development of professional associations and their
"organizational field" are so important to strategic adaptation,
we devote detailed attention to this topic in Chapter Seven.

Collective Goals

As described at the beginning of this chapter, professionals and
their associations pursue a wide variety of goals. Since strategies are undertaken to reach goals, if we wish to analyze the
strategies of professions we must make some simplifying assumptions about the nature of their goals. Based on the history of
health professions in the twentieth-century United States, we
posit two basic goals at the level of the professional community:
the achievement of legitimacy and market power.

   Legitimacy is the degree to which the profession's activities are consistent with the values of society. External stakeholders, particularly regulators and buyers, hold certain expectations for professions. Meeting these expectations is prerequisite
to being allowed to function as a profession. *Market power* is the
relative strength of practicing professionals in relationships with
buyers, suppliers, and substitutes. In studying business firms,
Porter (1980) argues that five forces — the bargaining power of
buyers, the bargaining power of suppliers, the threat of substitute products or services, the threat of new entrants, and rivalry
among firms — shape the marketplace for a business firm. For
professions, the threat of new entrants and rivalry among practitioners are primarily handled as internal management issues,
and they will be addressed as such in Chapter Seven. Buyers
and suppliers hold market power over professionals if they can
control the outcomes of their market exchanges with them, such
as the conditions of employment, prices of services, and prices
of inputs. To the extent that substitutes exist, professionals hold
less power in their exchanges with buyers and suppliers. Prac-

ticing professionals in a community share the goal of achieving market power relative to their buyers, suppliers, and substitutes.

In assuming these two collective goals, legitimacy and market power, we recognize the self-interested nature of professionals' goals in the form of market power, as well as society's influence on professionals and society's constraints on the pursuit of market power. The quest for market power takes place within the constraints of society's tolerance, and overzealous pursuit can result in the *loss* of legitimacy and, ultimately, market power. Our concept of collective goals is broader than Feldstein's (1991, p. 213), who in his study of professional associations states that "for purposes of this discussion, it is assumed that the legislative goals of the association are maximization of the incomes of its current members. Although health professionals have many goals, income is the only goal that all the health professionals in an association have in common." A caveat: our assumptions apply specifically to professions in the twentieth-century United States; that is, collective professional goals may vary from society to society.

Strategies

Strategic adaptation, as defined in Chapter One, is the process whereby professions shift their strategies in response to new demands from the environment. Strategies position the profession in relation to external demands. While professions are more loosely coupled than business firms, the notion that professional communities have strategies is consistent with new conceptualizations of business organizations.

In today's business world, many of the organizations are not traditional firms but loosely coupled collectives with a long-term strategic purpose. These have been referred to as quasi-firms, hybrids, networks, strategic alliances, and the like (Jarillo, 1988; Luke, Begun, and Pointer, 1989; Powell, 1987; Zuckerman and Kaluzny, 1991). As conceptualizations of the traditional business firm are becoming broader, they now encompass loosely coupled international firms and such entities as accounting partnerships and legal firms. Ghoshal and Bartlett

(1990, p. 603), for example, conceptualize the multinational corporation as an "inter-organizational network that is embedded in an external network consisting of all other organizations such as customers, suppliers, regulators, and so on, with which the different units of the multinational must interact." Astley and Brahm (1989) speak of the movement toward interorganizational modes of coordination among businesses as the economy shifts toward a high-technology base and global competition grows more intense. The fact that these collectives are loosely coupled does not reduce their ability to produce shared strategic activity, often referred to as collective strategy (Dollinger, 1990).

Earlier we argued that professional communities pursue market power and legitimacy as business organizations do. They also must be deeply concerned with a third arena of strategic decisionmaking—internal organization and management. While the remaining chapters delineate specific strategies for each of these arenas, here we introduce the general nature of those strategies.

Strategies for Legitimacy

The pursuit of legitimacy involves relating to the institutional environment—the "rules and requirements to which individual organizations must conform in order to receive legitimacy and support" (Scott, 1992, p. 132). These rules are created and enforced by courts, legislatures, buyer organizations, and other stakeholders. Conformity is accomplished primarily through *bridging* strategies, whereby organizations acquire approved types of personnel and develop "structural arrangements and production processes that conform to the specifications of established norms and/or authorities" (Scott and Meyer, 1991, p. 125).

Strategies for Market Power

Strategies to achieve market power primarily require shaping and managing relationships with three sets of stakeholders: buyers, suppliers, and substitutes. Like the quest for legitimacy, the pursuit of market power often requires bridging strategies

that increase the degree of coordination between exchange part-
ners (Pfeffer and Salancik, 1978). For organizations, bridging
strategies in the marketplace include bargaining, contracting,
cooptation, joint ventures, mergers, associations, and government connections (Scott, 1992).

Bridging strategies include what is often labeled vertical
integration. Vertical integration in business firms refers to the
incorporation of suppliers of inputs or distributors of outputs
into a focal production firm. An argument for vertical integration exists if an organization finds itself in a dependent relationship over which it seeks more control (Pfeffer and Salancik,
1978). Essentially, the external threat is reduced by internaliz-
ing and controlling it.

In professional communities, opportunities for vertical integration or forms of bridging are particularly prominent. One
option is to incorporate educators and educational institutions
as suppliers of new entrants to the professional community. A
second opportunity for linkage involves the suppliers of new
knowledge to the profession — research organizations and researchers. A third arena for integration is with regulators and
regulatory agencies — the stage agencies assigned the responsibility of controlling entry and regulating practice.

Bargaining is classified as a bridging strategy by Scott
(1992). Bargaining is likely to be a key strategy for health professions in the new environment, an option we discuss under the
rubric of *countervailing power*. As described by Galbraith (1980,
p. 111), the theory of countervailing power describes a process
whereby "economic power is held in check by the countervailing
power of those who are subject to it. The first begets the second."
To bargain with strong, organized buyer groups, for instance,
physicians must develop countervailing power (Light, 1991a).
While countervailing power can be developed in many different ways, we will emphasize building it through organization.

Another set of strategies relates mainly to establishing the
professional community's market power in relation to substitutes. In the broadest terms, these strategies involve bridging
with substitutes, competing with them, or diversifying the profession's work domain. Diversification requires the integration of

a new knowledge base into the profession, thrusting the professional community into a new set of stakeholder relationships.

Strategies for Internal Organization and Management

The assumption that professions develop strategies to achieve legitimacy and market power is similar to classifications of strategic decision-making arenas for business organizations. But professional communities face a third strategic challenge due to their loose coupling: internal organization and management. A relatively high degree of internal cohesion is assured by the employment relationship, so internal organization is less a priority of the business firm. In the study of business organizations, issues of structural design and management often are treated separately from strategic issues, although there is a growing awareness of the strategic nature of business organizations' structures (Powell, 1992). Because professional communities are so loosely structured, issues of internal organization and management assume the importance of other strategic issues.

Thus a third arena of strategic decision making is internal organization. Strategies for internal organization and management are directed at internal stakeholders—the individuals and associations that comprise the professional community. Internal issues are an important component of strategic adaptation for two reasons: internal structures must be aligned with environmental demands, and some degree of integration of the profession's loosely coupled elements is necessary if it is to function as a collective. Strategies for internal organization and management involve manipulating such elements as the size, knowledge base, culture, and organization of the community. Often the strategies are a form of bridging in that differentiated segments of the community are integrated with one another.

All three strategic decision-making arenas are interrelated. To attain market power and legitimacy requires appropriate internal organization and management. Success in achieving legitimacy can contribute to strength in the competitive arena and vice versa. Strategies in the different arenas may, however, conflict with each other. Strategies to upgrade entry educational credentials may satisfy legitimacy concerns, for example, but ignore demands of buyer organizations that professionals should be educated at the lowest possible cost. Successful organizations balance these conflicting demands from the environment while simultaneously managing their internal structures (Miles and Snow, 1978). Successful professional communities do the same.

Conventional and Contemporary Strategies

In the coming chapters, we distinguish between "conventional" and "contemporary" strategies of the health professions. Conventional strategies are those that have led to successful strategic adaptation in the United States in the twentieth century. Contemporary strategies, on the other hand, recognize the changing influence of external stakeholders on the strategies of the health professions. We argue that contemporary strategies are more likely to result in strategic adaptation of the health professions in the new environment and that, on balance, professions should shift their emphasis toward contemporary strategies.

Summary of the Framework

Figure 2.1 depicts the framework for strategic adaptation described thus far. Professional communities, comprised of individual professionals and their associations, engage in relationships with four key external stakeholders: buyers, suppliers, regulators, and substitutes. We differentiate one additional set of suppliers — teachers and researchers — as interface or internal stakeholders because most professions successfully incorporate teachers and researchers (but not other suppliers) within the professional community.

Relationships with these stakeholders are affected by the changing conditions sketched in Chapter One. Also influenced by these conditions is the internal structure of the profession, characterized by the professional community's size, composition, differentiation, knowledge base, organization, culture, and goals. The boundaries of the community are depicted by a wavy, permeable line indicating that potentially external stakeholders (particularly teachers and researchers but also regulators) may

Figure 2.1. A Framework for Strategic Adaptation.

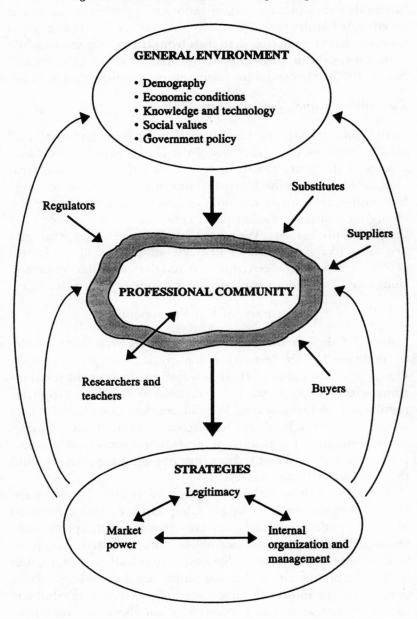

be integrated into the professional community. Therefore the community's boundaries are flexible.

In order to reach the shared goals of practitioners and their associations, professional communities develop plans and activities in the arenas of legitimacy, market power, and internal organization and management. The strategies in these three interrelated arenas determine the level of strategic adaptation achieved by the profession.

Also depicted in Figure 2.1 is the assumption that professional communities, through strategic activities, can influence conditions in both their task and general environments. Particularly, the strategies they use to manage their relationships with suppliers, buyers, regulators, and substitutes — stakeholders in the task environment — can change the general environment. Recognition of this possibility makes this a "strategic choice" rather than an "inertia" perspective (Shortell, Morrison, and Friedman, 1990) or a voluntaristic perspective more than a deterministic one (Astley and Van de Ven, 1983; Hrebiniak and Joyce, 1985). We recognize the constraining influence of environmental forces beyond the control of professions in shaping their strategies. For example, new technologies and new knowledge emanating from outside a professional community can lead to the development of substitutes for a profession's service and the demise of its buyer base. At the same time, professions are rarely helpless in the face of change. Through relationships with educational and research organizations, for instance, the professional community can influence the development of new knowledge and the emergence of new technologies that will directly affect its work domain. New markets can be sought to offset declines in the existing market; new product or service offerings can be created. We will emphasize the possibilities for strategic choice that professions face.

In Part Two of the book we elaborate the specific strategies used by professions to create legitimacy, achieve market power, and manage their internal dimensions. Yet the situation of each health profession is unique, as each has its own internal structure and its own set of relationships with interface and external stakeholders. In Part Three, we assess the past and future strategic adaptation of five different health professions.

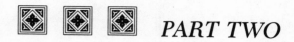 *PART TWO*

From Conventional to Contemporary Strategies

Chapter Three

Achieving and Maintaining Legitimacy

A major influence on a health profession's position relative to its stakeholders is the achievement of social legitimacy. The establishment of legitimacy is essential for the profession's claim to a specific work domain. In the twentieth century, achievement of legitimacy has largely involved the association of health professions with two basic values: scientific knowledge and health. The profession's claim that it contributes to health gives it an immediate and compelling rationale in the eyes of consumers, while the application of scientific knowledge has been the accepted pathway to achieving health. Today, however, social values such as access and efficacy of services are creating new requirements for legitimacy in the health professions, as is the growing challenge to the assumption that professionals' services really are based on scientific knowledge. Before exploring conventional and contemporary strategies for achieving legitimacy, we establish some basic working concepts.

The Concept of Legitimacy

In the marketplace, legitimacy depends on the acceptability or unacceptability of the business firm, its methods, and its output.

55

Acceptance or rejection is extended by stakeholders in the task environment and is based on an evaluative judgment rooted in deeply held values. Stakeholders may be the suppliers, substitutes, regulators, and buyers with which the firm interacts or subsets of these categories. Acceptance of a firm and its activities as "proper" entails an extension of credibility and respectability; rejection brings discredit and disrepute.

Legitimacy is crucial because a firm depends on the task environment for resources. Without credibility, these resources are threatened — a condition that ultimately can jeopardize the firm's survival. The claim that cigarette smoking is injurious to health, for example, a basic value, has caused legitimacy problems for tobacco companies and has seriously affected their domestic sales volume. On the other hand, the application of a "dolphin seal" on tuna cans by some tuna companies is an attempt to retain legitimacy by showing that their fishing processes do not violate environmental preservation values by putting dolphins at risk.

Like business firms, health professions must legitimate both *what* they do and *how* they do it. Health professions justify *what* they do by claiming that their activities contribute to health, a strongly held value. The credibility of the claim is linked to the efficacy of the profession's work. Within the constraints of current knowledge, if "health" is not forthcoming (on the average) from the actions of a health profession, then buyers would ultimately have no reason to continue patronizing it. In the twentieth century, *how* a health profession produces health has been legitimated by linking the profession's work to another strongly held value in our culture: science. Members of health professions presumably are educated in scientific knowledge, which is accepted by most stakeholders as the most powerful way of understanding the biochemical processes that influence the relative health of the human body. Education in scientific knowledge and work activities is intended to establish competence to perform the work. In turn, competence suggests that the actions will not be injurious but instead will contribute to the fundamental value: health.

An analysis of values in the legitimation of health professions should acknowledge several complexities. First, health professions seek legitimacy from a variety of stakeholders — ranging from individual consumers to organizations such as hospitals, insurance companies, HMOs, nursing homes, governments, and other health professions. Second, a variety of values are important in the legitimation considerations of stakeholders. While science and health remain important values, the current health care system has witnessed the rise of access, efficacy, and efficiency as salient values for legitimation. Third, the values are sometimes inconsistent — a condition highlighted by the current demand for high-quality health care and lower health care costs. A final complexity concerns the fact that legitimacy can vary in its breadth and depth. Ideally, a health profession wants recognition from a wide variety of stakeholders in its environment (breadth), as well as strong acceptance by these stakeholders (depth). The medical profession has been most successful in attaining this condition. Other health professions have had more limited success due to doubts arising from such values as science and efficiency.

Health professions must develop legitimation rationales which demonstrate that they share the values of key stakeholders. But legitimacy is not a static condition. Legitimation is a process requiring that health professions continually adapt to the changing universe of stakeholders as well as their changing and often conflicting values. The process may also require that a health profession understand the limitations on the breadth and depth of its legitimacy or evaluate the reasons for its loss or gain of legitimacy. In essence, legitimacy is a continuing problem for health professions, one that requires their continuing attention.

In the following discussion, we examine strategies that health professions can use in their efforts to gain legitimacy. At a high level of abstraction, all of the strategies involve bridging — linking the professional community to important stakeholders in its environment. The analysis describes specific strategies that have been used by health professions to attain recognition for the competence of their members, acceptance from organized buyers, and support for teaching and research from the government. Since the scientific training of health professionals is such an important source of legitimacy to most stakeholders within the task environment, particular attention is given to the matter of credentialing of the education and training process.

Credentialing Strategies

In the broadest sense, credentialing is the "formal recognition of professional or technical competence" (U.S. Department of Health, Education, and Welfare, 1976, p. 1). Its importance to legitimation arises because stakeholders of health professions, whether individual consumers or organizations, want health professionals to possess the competence to perform their work. Since a profession's claim of competence usually is based on an indication that its members have been trained in a formal body of knowledge that provides the basis for creditable performance, a basic legitimation strategy for a professional community in health care has been to construct a credentialing system. The system validates to buyers and regulators that the profession's members indeed possess training in formal knowledge. Formal knowledge, or higher knowledge, is knowledge that has been "formalized into theories and other abstractions, on efforts at systematic, reasoned explanation, and on justification of the facts and activities believed to constitute the world" (Freidson, 1986, p. 3). While formal knowledge need not be scientific, the two have been closely related in the United States and we will use formal knowledge and scientific knowledge interchangeably. (The same close relationship exists in other professions in the United States, as well — see Derber, Schwartz, and Magrass, 1990, pp. 27–35.) Basically, a credentialing system has communicated a health profession's identification with science, a key value in gaining legitimacy from most stakeholders.

A credentialing system involves a complex set of processes that often are interrelated. Individual members of a health profession are legitimated through the degrees and certificates granted by educational institutions, as well as certification, registration, and licensure by governmental or voluntary agencies. Another process, accreditation, involves a determination that an institution or program of study has met the quality standards established by some organization. Once the institution or program itself is legitimated, this reinforces the credibility of its products—the students. Since a credential (a degree or certificate) from an accredited institution or program often is required for certification or licensure, a relationship exists between organizational and individual credentialing. The credentialing process thus involves three basic types of organized stakeholders—educational sites, accreditation agencies, and government institutions—with whom health professions must deal in order to attain legitimacy through credentialing. As credentialing is a broad strategy, we next discuss specific strategies for dealing with each of these stakeholders.

Entry Education Credentials

Educational and training sites generally can be divided into two broad categories: academic institutions and nonacademic sites (for example, hospitals). In light of their well-established credibility in our society, formally recognized academic institutions usually lend greater legitimacy for the *initial* education of health professionals than nonacademic sites. Nonacademic sites usually have more legitimacy for later or postgraduate training *after* acquisition of the knowledge base or initial credential. Upon completion of the training at either site, a person usually receives some form of credential such as a degree, diploma, or certificate. The credential symbolically validates to society that the person is competent in the specified skills due to the successful completion of the educational program.

Site of Entry Education

As noted above, formally recognized educational institutions confer great legitimacy on the education of members of health professions. While establishing an educational program in a separate school within a university is particularly prestigious, gaining entry to such a setting is influenced strongly by two dimensions of the profession's knowledge base—its conventionality and complexity. "Conventional" or "orthodox" or "mainstream" knowledge is scientific medicine, which emphasizes biophysical science and somatic variables in order to understand disease. Using such disciplines as biology, chemistry, and physics, scientific medicine has gained widespread acceptance. The character of unorthodox knowledge typically varies from profession to profession. The chiropractic profession, for example, emphasizes that "normal transmission and expression of nerve energy are essential to the restoration and maintenance of health" (Maykovich, 1980, p. 307). Generally, gaining legitimacy within a university setting requires an orthodox knowledge base, one based upon scientific medicine.

Orthodox knowledge, however, does not assure a separate school within a university for a health profession. The complexity of knowledge — that is, its degree of abstraction — also affects this determination. A knowledge base grounded in complex scientific theory usually means that the academic members of the profession can pursue a significant research agenda. Since the generation of new knowledge through research is a major university goal, the profession is better positioned to legitimate its claim to a separate school than a health profession that lacks a foundation of complex knowledge. Allopathic medicine (MDs), pharmacy, and dentistry are the foremost examples of this logic.

Educational programs for health professions that lack a complex, orthodox knowledge base are more likely to be located in a variety of educational and training sites. If the sites are in a university setting, they are likely to have "program" status rather than a separate school. Educational programs for health services administrators may be situated in any of an extensive variety of sites within universities — schools of business, public health, allied health, and medicine, for example. Training also is more likely to occur in nonuniversity sites such as community colleges or nonacademic settings. Registered nurses exemplify this kind of "mixed" training site. Some registered nurse education occurs at separate schools in universities, but more new graduates come from community colleges. Although vastly reduced in number, some programs are located in a nonacademic setting: the hospital.

The example of registered nurse education highlights that

there are many types of *academic* institutions, a condition depicted by the Carnegie Classification of Institutional Type. Gaining legitimacy for a health profession's training program in an academic institution that is not a university typically involves emphasizing a value other than research. Specifically, many of these institutions emphasize training people to fill occupational roles demanded by society, so legitimating a curriculum means that a health profession must demonstrate a social need for the people trained in the particular work. Presumably such a demand can be translated into student enrollment, a prerequisite for a viable program. A university-based school or program that educates members of a health profession must address social needs as well, but there also is a greater emphasis on research than occurs at, say, community colleges.

Gaining legitimacy from a nonacademic educational or training site for a health profession typically involves different values, depending on the site. Nurse training programs located in hospitals, for example, were often a by-product of hospitals' continuing need for people trained in nursing skills. Profit is another example of a legitimizing value. Entrepreneurs have opened training programs for certain health auxiliaries in order to meet the market demand for health occupations with less complex knowledge bases.

In light of the foregoing discussion, several strategic considerations for health professions arise. First, since a health profession with an orthodox knowledge base has greater legitimacy with traditional academic sites, a health profession with an unorthodox knowledge base may opt for an independent strategy—bypassing the formal educational establishment and creating a separate institution. In the face of their rejection by the establishment, chiropractic and osteopathy followed this strategy in an effort to gain the legitimation of educational credentials for their practitioners. While an independent strategy assures the credentialing of its practitioners, the legitimacy of the credential to society at large, particularly consumers, remains an issue. Acquiring a credential from the educational establishment is desirable because such an institution validates education based on science, a value held in lofty esteem by society. The independent strategy means that the practitioner has a credential, but the education may not be rooted in mainstream science. The result is that the social legitimacy of such health professions is typically more narrow and shallow than that of professions based on orthodox knowledge. As we shall see in Chapter Four, competitors have attacked health professions with an unorthodox knowledge base as "quacks" in an effort to undermine their viability in the market. On the other hand, to the extent that market success is determined by efficacy of services and patient satisfaction, unorthodox health professions can be quite successful at achieving market power — witness the success of chiropractic (Wardwell, 1992).

Another strategic alternative for an unorthodox health profession is to become more conventional. Assimilation of orthodox knowledge is logical for a health profession, especially if it enhances legitimacy. This logic suggests a merger strategy — the knowledge bases of two health professions offering similar services become so similar that a merger of the professions appears an ultimate solution. Osteopathy and mainstream (allopathic) medicine are an example of this situation. In 1970, a college of osteopathy was established at a university (Michigan State) for the first time, and the medical and osteopathic colleges jointly shared the basic science departments. While debate about the distinctions between the two professions continues, it is clear that the growing similarity of their respective knowledge bases has contributed to a reduction in their distinctiveness (Wolinsky, 1988). The trend may enhance the acceptance of osteopathy in establishment educational institutions, but the profession must consider whether it ultimately is willing to sacrifice its identity as an autonomous profession.

Changes in the relative utility of science as a legitimating value suggest that affiliation with research-based universities may become less critical as a means of legitimating health professions. The ability of the profession's knowledge base to generate efficient, accessible, and efficacious treatment is increasingly important as well. In this respect, professions with unconventional knowledge bases and a diversity of entry education sites, including sites outside academia, may find themselves in less disadvantaged positions with regard to social legitimacy. Professions that are not cloistered in research-oriented universities will be better able to argue that they can meet society's needs for efficient, efficacious, and accessible services.

Complexity of Knowledge Base

For health professions that are based on conventional knowledge, a complex knowledge base has been an important way to enhance legitimacy. Professions typically have striven to develop a more substantial, abstract body of knowledge in order to enhance their legitimacy with universities. Most often, development of a more complex knowledge base is coupled with an increase in the length of the educational program. Many leaders in nursing advocate a baccalaureate program for educating registered nurses, for example, an approach that entails increasing the complexity of the knowledge base for nursing because it emphasizes "the theory and knowledge of how and why a particular disease receives a certain treatment" (Wolinsky, 1988, p. 273). This approach is designed to accelerate the shift of nurse training away from hospitals and community colleges to university programs.

In order to increase complexity, health professions can pursue two basic strategies: developing knowledge or pirating knowledge. In a development strategy, a health profession attempts to build its own complex, distinctive body of theoretical knowledge. The knowledge becomes the basis for educating practitioners in the profession's unique approach to a particular set of health problems. As described later in this chapter, another strategy — solicitation of government aid for research — is a complementary element of the development strategy. Nursing currently is struggling to develop a more complex and distinct knowledge base, and an Institute of Medicine (1989) study has suggested that certain allied health professionals must do the same in order to maintain their legitimacy in the university setting.

In contrast to the development strategy, a health profession could pursue a pirating strategy. In this approach, a profession exploits the knowledge base of another profession. Of course, extensive pirating would create increasingly similar professions, making a merger the ultimate implication. Pirating is likely to be incremental in nature, however, due to academic politics and the desire of most practitioners for their profession to retain a distinctive identity. Health care administration, for example, faces a continuing dilemma over how much to "borrow" from the disciplinary base of general business administration versus developing a distinctive disciplinary base of its own. Optometry's recent success in attaining the right to use diagnostic and therapeutic drugs, a right historically monopolized by physicians, exemplifies the pirating strategy. In legitimizing their competency to use drugs, optometrists emphasized that their educational curriculum concerning pharmaceuticals and vision care essentially embodied the same knowledge received by physicians. Indeed, their instructors were often physicians and pharmacists, the traditional sources of mainstream knowledge in this area of health care. Since the Pennsylvania College of Optometry is an independent institution, it was able to include education in pharmaceuticals in its curriculum without the resistance from the academic medical community that was encountered by optometry schools in universities with medical schools (Begun and Lippincott, 1980). As in this example, the pirating strategy usually occurs between two professions with orthodox knowledge bases because similarities in their intellectual foundation make the transfer of knowledge relatively easy. This does not foreclose the possibility of pirating between professions with orthodox and unorthodox knowledge bases, however. Mainstream physicians, for example, may use some of the techniques developed by chiropractic.

Enhancing the complexity of a knowledge base is a less attractive strategy for health professions today for several reasons. As professions compete more energetically for patients, the effort may encounter more than usual resistance from competitor professions threatened by intrusion on their turf. The competitors thus will likely oppose curriculum changes, arguing that the additional knowledge is duplicative, not distinctive. The profession seeking to enhance the complexity of its knowledge base, however, may be able to counter that the duplication will benefit consumers by increasing competition. Physical therapists used this argument relative to physicians for enhancing their entry level credentials beyond the baccalaureate.

But there is a greater problem with efforts to enhance the complexity of a health profession's knowledge base: the efforts may be perceived as an artificial attempt to inflate the profession's education beyond the skills required by its work domain. In addition to academic resistance, this charge may form the basis for opposition in the nonacademic environment. For example, a 1974 resolution by the New York Nurses' Association to require a baccalaureate degree in nursing as a condition of licensure was opposed as "incredibly costly," particularly in the absence of gains in quality or productivity that might justify the costs (Dolan, 1978). The incident demonstrates how new values in the health system can set constraints on the efforts by health professionals to legitimate themselves through increasing their credentialing standards.

Apart from its possible artificiality, a related problem with increasing the complexity of a profession's knowledge base concerns efficacy. A profession may increase the complexity of its knowledge base in an effort to enhance its legitimacy, only to encounter skepticism about the actual utility of the knowledge. A profession's knowledge base can become so complex that assessing the effectiveness of the profession's services is extremely difficult. If complexity is not accompanied by results, skepticism about its efficacy undermines the desired legitimacy. The psychiatric specialty within the medical profession is sometimes the object of such skepticism.

A final problem can arise from increasing the complexity of knowledge: it may induce cleavages within the profession. Members may balk at the push for upgraded credentials, as many practicing pharmacists are doing with reference to increasing the length of entry-level pharmacist education. Differences in education and training may become the basis for status differences within the profession, members with the more complex education presumably having superior status. The American Nurses' Association, for example, declared that registered nurses from baccalaureate programs would have a "professional" status while associate degree program graduates would have a "technical" status. This distinction gives rise to a schism within nursing, as nurses with the "technical" status, who form approximately two-thirds of the profession, have resisted the inferior designation (Wolinsky, 1988).

In summary, then, the strategy of increasing the complexity of the profession's knowledge base, while historically successful, is less likely to work today. In fact, many external stakeholders would reward movement in the opposite direction—toward reducing the length of training and therefore the educational costs and ultimately (perhaps) the price of services. Thus proposals for reducing the length of MD and other education may enhance the legitimacy of the profession on the grounds that they link the profession with values that are increasingly important to consumers, insurers, employers, and other external stakeholders. Opportunities to incorporate new educational technologies into curricula and develop more efficient educational processes, such as off-campus programs utilizing computer conferencing or teleconferencing technologies, exist in all the health professions. Innovative professions will push for the development of more efficient educational processes in the years ahead.

Accreditation of Educational Sites

Another set of strategic relationships concerns accrediting the institutions and programs that educate members of the health professions. Historically, the basic assumption has been that institutions or programs which meet standards concerning such matters as curriculum content, faculty degrees, laboratory equipment, and student-faculty ratios can be expected to produce competent graduates. By validating the institution or program, buyers are protected from the incompetence that might arise from the irregular educational sites mentioned earlier. Incentives for educational programs to seek accreditation generally are linked to posteducational credentialing; that is, licensure laws and private certification may require graduation from an accredited school or program. Even in the absence of such incentives, employers may still reward graduation from an accredited program by offering jobs to its graduates over graduates of nonaccredited programs.

Most accrediting agencies are created by professional associations, sometimes in concert with related organizations (Wilson and Neuhauser, 1985). The accrediting agency develops the accrediting standards while the U.S. Department of Education legitimates their activities by extending recognition to the accrediting agency (American Council on Education, 1991; Jonas and others, 1981). The primary accrediting agencies for twenty-six health professions are listed in Table 3.1. One agency, the Committee on Allied Health Education and Accreditation (CAHEA) of the American Medical Association, is responsible for accreditation of programs in six of the twenty-six professions. In each case, CAHEA collaborates with the profession's primary association. CAHEA ceases operating at the end of 1993, its activities superceded by individual accrediting agencies.

Gaining acceptance for an accreditation process from the federal government involves what Finkin calls the "reliance-recognition" approach. A prospective accrediting agency must gain the recognition of "the related academic and educational community" (Finkin, 1973, p. 372) before the government will legitimate an organization as an official accrediting agency. A prospective agency must demonstrate that its educational standards have gained broad acceptance in the educational community by persuading a significant number of the programs to accept the agency's standards.

Health professions have pursued program accreditation independently or in concert with a dominant profession. There are several accreditation strategies. First, a profession can control its own accreditation by developing an accrediting agency as an adjunct of its primary professional association. In this independent strategy, the professional association largely determines the standards of the educational institutions. The medical profession established this model, and it has been imitated by many of the so-called independent health professions (optometry, chiropractic, podiatry), as well as health care administration.

A second strategy makes use of the prevailing occupational

Table 3.1. Accrediting Organizations
for Entry-Level Education Programs: 1990.

Profession	Accrediting organization
Administrators, health care	Accrediting Commission on Education for Health Services Administration
Administrators, long-term care	none
Chiropractors	Council on Chiropractic Education
Dental hygienists	American Dental Association
Dental lab technicians	American Dental Association
Dentists	American Dental Association
Dietitians	American Dietetic Association
Medical record administrators	Committee on Allied Health Education and Accreditation — American Medical Association (CAHEA)
Medical technologists	CAHEA
Nurse anesthetists	Council of Accreditation of Nurse Anesthesia Educational Programs — American Association of Nurse Anesthetists
Nurse-midwives	American College of Nurse-Midwives
Nurses, registered	National League for Nursing
Occupational therapists	CAHEA
Optometrists	American Optometric Association
Pharmacists	American Council on Pharmaceutical Education
Physical therapists	American Physical Therapy Association
Physician assistants	CAHEA
Physicians — DOs	American Osteopathic Association
Physicians — MDs	Liaison Committee on Medical Education — American Medical Association and Association of American Medical Colleges
Podiatrists	American Podiatric Medical Association
Psychologists	American Psychological Association
Radiologic technologists	CAHEA
Recreational therapists	Council on Accreditation — National Therapeutic Recreation Society and National Recreation and Park Association
Repiratory therapists	CAHEA
Social workers, medical	Council on Social Work Education
Speech-language pathologists and audiologists	American Speech-Language-Hearing Association

Source: American Council on Education, 1991; American Medical Association, 1990a; Association of University Programs in Health Administration, 1991; Stanfield, 1990; U.S. Department of Health, Education, and Welfare, 1977b; U.S. Department of Health and Human Services, 1992; Wardwell, 1992.

structure of the health care system. A clinical health profession, for instance, may seek formal approval from the American Medical Association, which uses guidelines to determine whether recognition is appropriate for the emerging profession. The most important consideration is whether a "failure or omission" in the occupational structure justifies a new occupation (Lazarus, Levine, and Lewin, 1981). Substantive educational requirements (the "essentials"), defining what the new practitioners should be qualified and trained to do, are developed with the collaboration of the AMA and interested allied health occupations and medical specialties. The AMA's Council on Medical Education has final approval authority over the essentials, while CAHEA accredits the allied health education program. Essentially, then, a health profession derives legitimacy within the health care system by first seeking approval from the dominant independent profession. Although there is a loss in market power that follows from subordination, these sacrifices are made on the assumption that legitimacy is gained from the sanction of the dominant profession.

A third strategy — rebellion — is an outgrowth of the foregoing strategy. A health profession may begin by getting the sanction of a dominant profession, but after becoming established it may rebel and seek independent accreditation. An example is physical therapy. Physical therapy was established and recognized by the AMA in 1936, but disagreements erupted between the medical community and physical therapy concerning referrals, department directorships, and authority over treatment plans. In the late 1970s, the American Physical Therapy Association (APTA) withdrew from its collaborative relationship with the AMA and sought the independent right to accredit physical therapy programs. After a period in which APTA and CAHEA each accredited physical therapy programs, APTA established independent control. Occupational therapy is likely to follow this strategy, as well.

Whatever the approach — independence, dependence, or rebellion — the strategy of accrediting educational programs is subject to important criticisms today. The possibility that accreditation can be used to control supply and stifle educational program innovation is particularly threatening to consumers, employers of health professionals, and other stakeholders. Events in the accreditation history of nursing offer an example. In 1965, the commissioner of the Office of Education approved the National League for Nursing (NLN) as the sole agency for accrediting nurse education. The junior college association and the American Hospital Association, however, felt that the NLN's specialized program accreditation, which was required in addition to accreditation by state and regional agencies, was too stringent: many programs were not being accredited, thus jeopardizing their involvement with educational assistance programs for nurses. Ultimately, the conflict was settled by federal legislation that effectively expanded accrediting authority to include reliance on state and organizational accreditation. In effect, there was a conflict between two legitimizing values: quality of care and access to care. Congress chose the latter value, thereby undercutting NLN's attempt to attain independence in accreditation.

Accrediting agencies today are considered by some stakeholders as protecting a small number of elite educational programs in order to keep supply down relative to demand. Accrediting criteria often include requirements that programs have a minimum length and a minimum number of faculty members. As an example, health care administration program accrediting criteria set a minimum length for programs (at least two academic years) and express a "belief" that a minimum of three full-time faculty are required (Accrediting Commission on Education for Health Services Administration, 1990). Thus innovative programs that may strive to convey knowledge in a shorter time period, or using part-time rather than full-time faculty, are handicapped in the accreditation process.

These concerns mean that health professions should be more careful to create accrediting bodies and program accreditation criteria that are responsive to demands of external stakeholders. In the past, internal stakeholders (practitioners) and interface stakeholders (teachers and researchers) have dominated accrediting bodies. In addition to creating some degree of independence from professional associations, accrediting agencies should expand their structures to involve these key stakeholders.

Postgraduate Credentialing

Although professionals usually receive a credential (degree or certificate) from the institution where they undertake their initial education, there is a third credentialing strategy: requiring health professionals to receive additional credentials. These credentials can be divided into two types—public regulation and private certification. Public regulation involves the public sector through government sanction. Private certification involves nongovernmental agencies, usually the professional associations of the health professions themselves or adjuncts of these associations.

Public Regulation

In general, public regulation as a credentialing strategy involves a profession developing and lobbying for a law that provides government recognition of the profession. The attempt to gain regulatory recognition usually involves making the case for protection of the "public health and safety" to a specific organized stakeholder—state political institutions. The health profession typically argues that regulation is necessary because consumers may lack knowledge about the nature and quality of the service needed, the competence of the practitioner rendering the service, and the quality of the service rendered.

While there are many possible modes of public regulation (Institute of Medicine, 1989), three basic options are available to health professions: licensure, registration, and certification. Licensure provides the greatest depth and breadth of legitimation because it entails exclusionary compulsion. Under force of state law, only a person with a license is allowed to practice the profession. The licensure law defines the practice domain of the profession—that is, the work whose performance requires possession of the license—as well as any conditions that attend the performance of the work. Licensure also usually involves a structure—a licensing board—that is often composed largely of members from the regulated profession. Licensing boards are legally authorized to perform such functions as establishing entry standards, promulgating practice standards and rules of professional conduct, and investigating and disciplining members of the profession.

It is important to establish the connection between this structure, the scientific knowledge that underlies most modern health professions, and the protection that it presumably offers buyers. Licensing board control over entry standards provides an example. As Moore (1961, p. 104) notes: "Licensing, it is argued, increases information by establishing minimum standards for entrants. In effect, all practitioners must meet certain minimum qualifications, for no unlicensed practitioners are permitted. The consumer therefore knows that practitioners of the licensed occupation possess a given degree of competence." The degree of competence is assured through entry barriers that are designed to establish that the prospective practitioner's competence is sufficient to pose no harm to buyers. The entry barriers usually include educational requirements, experience requirements (such as medical internship), and passage of a licensure exam. Since their knowledge presumably puts them in the best position to determine the entry standards and to evaluate whether candidates meet the standards, members of a health profession often are given control over public licensure functions.

Public certification and registration have traditionally provided less breadth and depth of legitimation than licensure. Certification means that the use of a particular occupational title is restricted to those who have obtained a formal certificate of competence from the state. Obtaining such a certificate — a voluntary action — is contingent on meeting specified standards (for example, an educational degree in the field) that have been advocated by the professional association. This form of regulation is weaker than licensure because it only forbids unauthorized use of the occupational *title* and does not exclude noncertified individuals from practicing the profession. Registration is an even weaker form of occupational control because it essentially involves a state agency recording a person's name, address, and education. It, too, is a voluntary action, but unlike licensure and certification a registration system usually does not require that people fulfill certain requirements, such as levels of education or experience. Evidence that the complexity of a health profession's knowledge base is associated with the form of regulatory sanction it receives from states (Graddy, 1989) suggests that professions lacking the complex knowledge to justify licensure often pursue the certification and registration options.

The public regulatory status of twenty-six health professions is given in Table 3.2. All twenty-six are regulated in some form in some states except health care administrators (although *public health department* administrators are regulated in four states). Seventeen of the twenty-six professions are separately regulated in more than forty states, demonstrating the extensiveness of public regulation of the health professions.

Public credentialing of health professionals, particularly credentialing by licensure, has come under increasing criticism from consumer groups, provider organizations, and insurers. Such criticisms include the charge that licensing boards protect rather than expose low-quality practitioners (Gross, 1984); that licensing laws inhibit innovation and competition and raise prices and reduce access to services (Young, 1987; Begun and Feldman, 1990); and that the credentials of professionals are symbolic rather than substantial, signifying the attainment of power but not ability (Collins, 1979). These criticisms strike at the core of legitimacy for the health professions — their commitment to people's health rather than the professional's interests.

As a strategy for legitimation, the creation of licensing statutes is of declining utility to the health professions owing to its negative effects on many powerful stakeholders. To respond to these developments, health professions can support reforms to make licensing laws more effective in achieving internal quality control of professional practice. They can support certification or registration of new professions, rather than licensing. They can implement greater outsider participation on regulatory boards. They can introduce more flexibility into current licensing laws — for instance, by allowing for overlapping boundaries of practice and multiple pathways for entry (Institute of Medicine, 1989).

Private Certification

Unlike licensure, credentialing through private certification is undertaken by a nongovernmental agency. Certification typically involves affirmation of initial education or recognition of

Table 3.2. State Regulation of Selected Health Professions: 1990

Profession	Number of States Licensing	Number of States Regulating[a]
Administrators, health care	50	50
Administrators, long-term care	0	0
Chiropractors	50	51
Dental hygienists	51	51
Dentists	51	51
Denturists	8	8
Dietitians	16	20
Medical record administrators	2	2
Medical technologists	6	9
Nurse anesthetists[b]	8	10
Nurse-midwives[b]	16	50
Nurses, registered	51	51
Occupational therapists	40	43
Optometrists	51	51
Pharmacists	51	51
Physical therapists	50	51
Physician assistants	23	49
Physicians — DOs	50	50
Physicians — MDs	51	51
Podiatrists	51	51
Psychologists	51	51
Radiologic technologists	21	27
Recreational therapists	2	4
Respiratory therapists	13	24
Social workers, medical	42	47
Speech-language pathologists and audiologists	41	42

[a]Registration, certification, or licensure.
[b]Also regulated as registered nurses if no separate regulation exists.
Source: Data for administrators from Stanfield, 1990, p. 355; all others compiled from Council of State Governments, 1990.

specialty training beyond an initial credential. Since private certification is controlled by professional associations, attainment of the credential may not provide legitimation to certain stakeholders. As we shall see, the extent of legitimacy achieved by private certification usually depends on its purpose.

Using a *specialty* strategy in private certification, practitioners seek specialized graduate training beyond their initial education. Often the training occurs outside an academic institution, such as a hospital where specialized technology is located. Since it indicates successful completion of specialized training, private certification often becomes the basis for distinguishing among practitioners who already hold similar basic credentials. The most elaborate example of this strategy is specialty recognition within the medical profession. Such recognition — essentially a form of accreditation — is made by the American Board of Medical Specialties (ABMS), which is composed of representatives of the existing specialty boards and the AMA. A prospective specialty can be granted either "primary" or "conjoint" status. The former indicates complete independence from existing specialties; the latter indicates a subordination to sponsors drawn from existing specialties. The key issue in the legitimation of a prospective specialty is whether there is a "justifiable need for the new category." But often the process involves a variety of considerations, including the politics surrounding the division of labor within the medical profession (Lazarus, Levine, and Lewin, 1981).

A physician receiving board certification from a legitimated specialty board will have the greatest legitimacy in the health care system, but to receive such legitimation, it is necessary to complete a residency program. The program usually is undertaken in a hospital that has been approved by the Accreditation Council for Graduate Medical Education. Following completion of a residency, the physician must pass a comprehensive examination developed and administered by the specialty board from whom certification is sought. Fulfillment of any additional requirements results in "board certification" in the specialty area. To retain the certification, the physician must meet any recertification guidelines established by the specialty board. The sanctioned status thus distinguishes the physician from peers who share common basic credentials — the medical degree and licensure.

There have been two major limitations to pursuing a specialty strategy through private certification. First, it is difficult to sanction those who claim an ability to perform the specialized skills but do not go through the certification process. The second problem is structural. While medicine certifies only twenty-three specialties through the ABMS, for instance, some eighty-six are listed on the AMA's annual questionnaire (Roback, Randolph, and Seidman, 1990). There is nothing to prevent these groups from forming "certification boards" independent of the ABMS, as many have.

The other basic type of private certification strategy is *affirmation*. Like the specialty strategy, affirmation entails a health professional association, or an organizational adjunct, legitimizing the competence of practitioners. It does not concern specialized training beyond the basic credentials, however; rather, the professional association affirms the basic training of prospective members of the profession. This type of legitimation has been categorized here as "certification," but it can assume other forms such as registration and association membership. That is, the granting of association membership or entry on the association's registry of "qualified" practitioners constitutes recognition of competence (U.S. Department of Health, Education, and Welfare, 1971).

There are two important subtypes of affirmation: broad and narrow. To achieve certification by a professional association typically means that a person must meet certain entry standards such as educational requirements, practice experience, examination, and association membership. These standards can be broad or narrow. Early in the development of a health profession, when there is a concern for gaining a critical mass of members, the entry conditions tend to be broad. Before 1987, for example, the certifying examination for physician assistants was open to those who had "informal" training, as well as graduates of physician assistant and nurse practitioner training programs. Beginning in 1987 the examination was closed to informal trainees and graduates of certain nurse practitioner programs. Evidently, physician assistants are adopting a narrow affirmation strategy, one which reflects a tightening of standards, particularly with regard to antecedent educational credentials.

Like public regulation, private certification strategies may have an adverse effect on key stakeholders of the health professions. Offered by the professional association itself—not some institution ostensibly separate from the professional community—

the credential may be perceived as artificial and may serve as a barrier to entry to specialized practice. Health professions will increasingly need to demonstrate that certified practitioners provide more efficacious or cost-effective care than noncertified practitioners if they are to convince stakeholders, such as insurers and employers, of the need for certification. Nurses certified or not certified in neonatal intensive care were recently the subject of one such study ("Study to Probe . . . ," 1990). If private certification is pursued, health professions can work with buyer groups, such as employers or consumer groups, to create certification systems that are more responsive to buyer needs and thus more legitimating for the profession.

In addition to credentialing, an important form of recognition in modern health care systems is society's willingness to provide resources to health professions. Acquisition of resources by the professional community increasingly requires links with organized buyers and government. Organized buyers control access to large numbers of clients, and government can support the expansion of research and teaching within the professional community. We turn now to the strategies used by health professions to gain these important resources.

Gaining Acceptance from Organized Buyers

Formal recognition by key buyers dramatically facilitates the overall acceptance of a health profession in society. Two important buyer organizations are hospitals and health insurers. Hospitals offer space and technological resources that can provide significant support for health professionals who practice independently, and they are the major employer of many health professionals. Given the hospital's importance in the health system, its acceptance of a profession through extending admitting privileges or employing credentialed professionals is a major source of legitimacy. Acceptance from health insurers is another importance source of legitimacy. As "third parties" have become the major source of funds that pay for health care in the United States, recognition of a health profession's services for reimbursement by insurers is another source of respectability. Further, recognition by one major insurer, such as Medicare, carries weight with other buyers, regulators, and stakeholders.

Hospital Privileges

Control over hospital privileges has long been dominated by the medical profession, and medicine has long been reluctant to extend privileges to nonphysician health professionals. Implicitly hospitals accepted the judgment of the physician community that nonphysician providers were of lower quality and that quality should be the primary value. Prior to 1985, interpretation of the accreditation manual of the Joint Commission on Accreditation of Hospitals (now the Joint Commission on Accreditation of Healthcare Organizations) allowed only physicians and dentists to be on the medical staff. Other categories of privileges, such as "limited practitioner with clinical privileges" and "specified professional personnel," also existed. The rationale for this rigorous control over the privilege system was to assure competent care by practitioners — a by-product of a historical past in which practitioners' competence (mainly among physicians) was a serious problem. Subordination of nonphysician practitioners (except dentists) in the hospital was derived from the logic that physicians' supervision of nonphysicians was a way to assure the quality of care provided by these practitioners.

In 1985, however, the JCAH manual changed the privilege standards. Essentially, granting medical staff membership and clinical privileges is now a matter for each hospital to determine. The new rationale for making such determinations includes such factors as the hospital's corporate mission, community needs, cost of services, quality of care, a justifiable expectation of the need to admit patients, appropriate moral character, major malpractice problems, and the ability to render care within his or her license. Whatever the grant of privileges (for instance, staff, clinical, or admitting) to nonphysicians, the JCAHO still requires physician evaluation of an admitted patient, as well as physician responsibility for the patient's general medical condition. Given the need for hospitals to broaden their patient base and to render efficient care, hospital boards and administrators are likely to become more receptive to extending privileges to nonphysician practitioners.

In light of the history of hospital privileges, an appeal to efficiency may be insufficient to gain hospital access. But nonphysicians might test whether the negative attitudes within the medical profession are really changing, a possibility that suggests one strategic option. A member of a nonphysician profession may pursue a "sponsor" strategy when a member of the medical staff is willing to support an application for hospital privileges. Such a strategy has been recommended to optometrists (Fisher, 1988). The strategy is designed to validate the applicant's application through the staff member's support and to provide an advocate who will address any issues that might arise during the process.

If the sponsor strategy fails, it may be necessary for nonphysician health professionals to seek legitimation for hospital privileges from an institution outside the hospital. A legal strategy — shifting the attempt to gain hospital privileges to the courts — is one possibility. The balance of power between physicians and nonphysicians is more equal in the courts than in hospitals, something that the psychology profession understands from its successful use of lawsuits to gain hospital privileges. Alternatively, a political strategy shifts the effort to gain legitimacy to state legislatures. State licensing statutes that regulate hospitals often include provisions concerning who holds hospital privileges. State laws frequently have reinforced the medical profession's domination of hospital privileges, but podiatrists have been successful in gaining clinical privileges through legislation. Successful use of these strategies means that a health profession must understand the specific values that can legitimate its claim in that arena. Psychology, for example, appealed to antitrust laws, which emphasize the value of a free market, in its effort to gain hospital privileges.

Gaining hospital privileges has great potential for broadening the legitimacy of nonmedical clinical professions. Staff privileges would certainly enhance the ability of nonmedical providers to challenge physicians as substitutes. "Conditioned" privileges would circumvent their historical exclusion, of course, but this situation would limit the competitive threat of the nonmedical professions. Access to admitting privileges would expand the target base of buyers of the provider's services.

Health Insurers

The legitimation of health professionals by another important organized buyer, health insurers, involves at least five different organized stakeholders. Two types of insurers — Medicaid (involving both state and federal government) and Medicare (involving the federal government) — are public in character, while three others (Blue Cross/Blue Shield, commercial companies, and HMOs) are private. Clearly, mainstream medicine has been the health profession most accepted by health insurers. The services of some health professions have been rejected for health insurance coverage. Others have encountered restrictive reimbursement provisions such as exclusions in the coverage of services provided by nonphysician professions, differential reimbursement rates, and procedural limitations on providing coverage (for example, requiring the presence of a physician). Health maintenance organizations probably have offered the most acceptance to nonphysician practitioners, although podiatrists and psychologists have complained about exclusion (Lazarus, Levine, and Lewin, 1981, p. V-25).

In the past, efforts by health professions to achieve legitimation in the eyes of health insurers involved discussion of one central value: quality. In their eyes, technical competence and the safety of procedures have been the major quality concerns regarding nonphysician practitioners. Insurers claim that these concerns have justified limitations on reimbursement for nonphysician professions. This situation reemphasizes the importance of the credentialing system as central to professional legitimation, for the educational credentials of its members are designed to validate their competence. In response, insurers sometimes claim that licensure laws are inadequate and establish only minimum standards. Nonphysician practitioners have used this charge to rationalize upgrading their credentials.

In the new health care environment, legitimation rationales concerning health insurers will pivot around the values of cost-effectiveness and efficacy. Insurers often want proof that nonphysician professionals indeed are more cost-effective than physicians and that the provision of insurance will not induce an increase in costs by these practitioners that would eliminate any cost differentials. Moreover, a major concern of insurers is whether the costs of nonphysician professionals are "controllable" — that is, whether the service is amenable to precise definition, to reasonable accuracy in estimation of occurrence, and to some kind of use limitation. In response to the uncertainty about the cost implications, insurers sometimes see excluding professions other than medicine as a way to control the unpredictability. Nonphysician practitioners thus are compelled to demonstrate that they are a cost-effective resource. Evidence about relative prices and quality is an appropriate response to these concerns.

Despite an appeal to cost-effectiveness and efficacy, nonphysician clinical health professions still may not attain recognition due to the influence of physicians' expertise and status in health insurance companies. As with hospital privileges, it may thus be necessary to pursue the sponsor, legal, or political strategies. Seeking sponsors within an insurer is a prudent strategy, but barring allies it is likely that nonphysician professions will have to shift their case to the legal or political arena. A telling example of the legal strategy is the successful suit that psychologists brought against Blue Shield over certain health insurance coverage issues (Lazarus, Levine, and Lewin, 1981).

Political strategies remain important because political institutions play a major role in determining what procedures are reimbursed and what conditions regulate the coverage of a profession's services. The federal government finances Medicare; the federal and state governments finance Medicaid; states have responsibility for the regulation of health insurers. Given the increasing importance of health care costs, efficiency is a key value in the legitimation efforts of nonphysician clinical professions in Medicare and Medicaid. It must be shown that the efficiencies will be "real" and will not entail a sacrifice of quality. At the state level, various nonphysician professions — including dentists, podiatrists, psychologists, and nurse-midwives — have gained inclusion in health insurance through state statutes. Freedom of choice, a consumer value long espoused by the medical profession, as well as claims of unfair discrimination, have figured prominently in these legitimation efforts.

In addition to these strategies, it is also possible to pursue a consumer-focused strategy. Using this strategy, a health profession actively develops support from consumer groups to pressure insurers. A coalition in a Pennsylvania community successfully lobbied a Blue Shield board, composed of a majority of physicians, to alter the terms of reimbursement for nurse-midwives (Lazarus, Levine, and Lewin, 1981). The entry of consumers into the deliberations about coverage injected two other important values into the debate: consumer preferences and access to care. While consumers can be an important ally in gaining legitimacy with health insurers, nonmedical clinical providers must address the fact that some consumers perceive nonmedical providers as providing a lower quality of care.

Because of the growing importance of cost-effectiveness as a legitimating value held by key stakeholders, even the health professions with considerable legitimacy are being forced to respond. The medical profession, as evidenced by a joint AMA–Rand Corporation research effort, for example, has begun collecting evidence that allows the medical community to identify more cost-effective treatments for certain conditions. Health professions can advance their strategic adaptation by moving vigorously to link their profession to the buyer's concern for cost-effective and efficacious care.

Gaining Government Support

Many of the health professions have benefited from the government's subsidization of research and education. Subsidization of research supports the development of the body of knowledge for educating and training health professionals; subsidization of education supports increasing the size of the health profession. In effect, this support builds the core of the professional community — its formal knowledge and the number of its practitioners.

Given the central role that formal knowledge plays in the legitimation of health professions through credentialing, it is logical for a health profession to legitimate itself further by gaining financial support from society for the development of formal knowledge through research. Biomedical research, both basic and applied, is a major means for generating the formal knowledge, technology, and equipment used by clinical health practitioners. The medical profession has been the primary recipient of support for biomedical research, much of it distributed through the National Institutes of Health (NIH). Using an external grant program — universities, medical schools, and affiliated teaching hospitals have been the principal recipients — NIH has focused on categorical diseases because of congressional mandates and the preferences of medical researchers. The categorical logic of the research allocations suggests the underlying rationale for such spending: its presumed contribution to "health" by facilitating the conquest of specific diseases such as cancer and heart disease. Moreover, some professions have been able to establish specific research funding. The National Center for Nursing Research, authorized in 1985 as part of NIH, is such an example: organized nursing "viewed authorization of the center as a milestone in the acceptance of nursing as a research-based profession" (Kovner, 1990, p. 100).

With regard to the terms of legitimacy, research spending has interesting ramifications. On its face, the medical profession has attained a legitimacy that simultaneously abets achievement of its other goals. A major consequence of research spending has been the rise of medical specialization, which has resulted in higher incomes and prestige for physicians trained in the specialties. This form of legitimation may have unintended consequences, however, for technology and specialization are prominent contributors to the health care cost crisis. If the cost problems ultimately prompt expanded government intervention in the health system, the effects on medicine's market power may be quite negative, as greater government control is likely to reduce medicine's power relative to buyers, regulators, and substitutes. Such intervention also has the potential for slowing the assimilation of high technology and specialized medicine by the health care system — an effect that would reduce any contributions of technology and specialization to the social welfare.

Recent declines in the growth of NIH funding, as well as the debate about the relative contribution of high-tech specialized medicine to health, may provide an opening for nonmedical professions to pursue a research legitimation strategy. Researchers in nursing, for example, have sought research support for investigating geriatric problems such as the causes of falls in the elderly and urinary incontinence. Such research clearly has the potential for an important contribution to social welfare, especially in light of ongoing demographic shifts. Likewise, allied health professions might attempt to legitimate support for developing their scientific base — a need highlighted by an Institute of Medicine study (1989) — by appealing to efficiency. If these professions can indeed contribute to efficient care in a time of high health care costs, they might have a viable case. A similar case can be made for research on prevention, health promotion, and alternative therapies (as opposed to new therapies based on the medical model).

Apart from support for research, it is logical for health professional communities to seek assistance for educating and training their members. By supporting an increase in the number of practitioners in a profession, society expresses its esteem for the profession. Unlike the support for research, subsidies for education have been more widely distributed, as noted in Chapter One. A number of health professions — dentistry, nursing, optometry, pharmacy, podiatry, and various allied health professions, as well as the medical profession — have received support for education.

The rationale for such support is important because it is an example of how values other than science increasingly influence legitimacy. At the time that legislation was passed to support health professional education, there was a perceived shortage of health care personnel. Since access to care, an important value in the health care system, was assumed to be positively correlated with the number of practitioners available to deliver care, this value strongly influenced political decisions on government support for educating health professionals. An additional assumption in providing such aid was that training these professionals in educational institutions would improve the quality of care. Of course, this rationale reflects the importance of identification with science in legitimizing modern health professions.

An analysis of the terms of legitimacy reveals different consequences for different health professions. The medical profession long resisted federal aid to medical education (Ginzberg, 1990), and the consequences of such aid (a larger supply of MDs) are potentially adverse for the profession's market power. A physician surplus creates potential for greater internal competition among physicians, greater competition with substitutes, and a relative power shift to buyers of physician services, since buyers can more easily shop for cheaper care. Moreover, a declining rate of return on medical education may signal diminishing attractiveness of the profession to prospective entrants.

Using the allied health professions as an example, however, reveals a different situation. Educational support for these professions contributes mainly to their status by helping to develop sufficient numbers of personnel so that the professions can establish a firm position in the health care system. An Institute of Medicine (1989) analysis suggests that this remains a problem for many allied health professions. As in the case of research support, these professions might consider arguing for continuing support for education due to the potential efficiency of their practitioners. Additionally, many of the nursing and allied health professionals are more likely than physicians to locate in underserved areas, thereby helping to increase access to care.

Enhancing Public Image

There are other methods that health professions use to bridge with important social values. Most common, probably, is the undertaking of large-scale public relations campaigns by professional associations to demonstrate the congruence of the profession's values with strongly held public values. Historically, these campaigns have involved efforts to present professionals as caring, service-oriented, high-quality providers. Such campaigns build internal esprit de corps and a reservoir of goodwill with external stakeholders that can be drawn upon as the profession strives for formal recognition in governmental and judicial settings.

We can expect that as stakeholders' demands for accessible and cost-effective care continue to build, health professions can strategically adapt by communicating how they are meeting these demands. The American Medical Association, for example, in 1991 funded a series of advertisements and dissemination of brochures on the topic of the service orientation of physicians. An advertisement noted that "over a quarter million AMA physicians are dedicated to providing medical care with compassion and respect for human dignity" and share a "concern about bringing quality health care to underserved groups" (from an untitled ad in *Newsweek,* Aug. 19, 1991). The public relations program reflected a strategic decision to link physicians to public values of quality (a value of traditional appeal) and access (a value of new appeal). Other associations, such as the American Nurses' Association, have publicized their endorsement of national health reforms to meet the needs of the uninsured as well as organized buyer groups.

Conventional and Contemporary Strategies

Health professions generally have been granted an unusual degree of legitimacy in the United States. They comprise the major portion of the occupations that have been granted self-regulation through state licensure, for instance. Health professions are rated among the highest in surveys of trust and respect of occupations. The identification of health professions with science and with the positive goal of health is seldom challenged.

The values under which most health professions originally achieved legitimacy are shifting, however, and it is critical that health professional communities recognize and respond to this shift in values. Stakeholders' values increasingly include cost-effectiveness, efficacy, and access. Besides, the link between the services of the health professions and "health" itself is increasingly being challenged and empirical evidence is being demanded.

Professional judgments about this linkage are no longer accepted by insurers, consumers, and other stakeholders.

In light of these changes, health professions must pursue more contemporary strategies in order to strategically adapt. Such a movement would encourage these professions to examine themselves with the same lens that external stakeholders are using. Table 3.3 summarizes the conventional and contemporary strategies for achieving and maintaining legitimacy.

Rather than following traditional pathways toward profession building—such as lengthening educational requirements and strictly controlling diversity in educational program cur-

Table 3.3. Strategies for Legitimacy.

Conventional Strategies

- Affiliate entry educational programs with research-oriented universities.
- Upgrade entry education by expanding complexity of the knowledge base.
- Develop strong control over accreditation of educational programs by the primary professional association.
- Seek public regulation through state licensing.
- Create private certification in response to internal pressures.
- Achieve hospital privileges and insurers' acceptance through legal or political channels or sponsorship by physicians.
- Base the rationale for research support from government on the treatment of specific diseases within the medical model.
- Enhance public image by emphasizing quality and service.

Contemporary Strategies

- Avoid cloistering of entry educational programs in research-oriented universities.
- Streamline entry education; keep its length as short as possible.
- Involve consumers, employers, and other external stakeholders in the educational program accreditation process.
- Seek a minimal form of public regulation or none at all. Introduce flexibility into existing licensing laws.
- Create private certification only in response to buyers' demands.
- Achieve hospital privileges and insurers' acceptance through development of empirical evidence of cost-effectiveness and efficacy. Form alliances with consumers.
- Base the rationale for research support from government on prevention of disease, health promotion, efficacy, and cost-effectiveness.
- Base the rationale for educational support from government on solving society's problems of access, cost, chronic disease, and the like.
- Enhance public image by emphasizing the contribution to lower costs and improved access.

---

ricula—professions may be better served by accommodating diversity and innovation in their educational programs. State and private credentialing of individual practitioners, rather than an internal system of reward and control, should be responsive to buyers' needs. And professions must demonstrate their responsiveness to the concerns of hospitals, organized buyers, government, and consumers by delivering cost-effective and efficacious services and promoting greater access to them.

Legitimation is an active process. Health professions should continue to be alert to the emergence of new stakeholders and their values, shifts from long-standing values, and the emergence of conflicting values.

Legitimacy provides the foundation for a health profession's long-term existence within the social system. Yet increasingly health professions must also prove themselves in the economic marketplace. Next we turn to strategies for achieving market power.

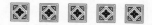

Chapter Four

Managing Relationships with Substitute Professions

As health care has become a more competitive industry in the United States, health professionals have found themselves in competition with practitioners from other professions, with consumer self-help, and with other forms of substitutes. Incentives for society to discover self-treatments and preventive measures for health problems are becoming more and more intense as health costs escalate. The efforts by major purchasers of health services to find cheaper substitutes will no doubt swell in intensity as well. These substitution risks are particularly imminent for the routine aspects of a profession's work. Robots, for example, can do some of the routine tasks of pharmacists. Consumers can choose eyeglasses by trial and error from drugstore displays.

This chapter examines the strategies used by health professions in their effort to manage relationships with other professions that offer substitute services. The traditional approach has been to monopolize a work domain or marginalize the tasks performed by substitutes. Even in those professions that have managed to establish monopolies, such as medicine and dentistry, challenges from substitutes are present and rising. Before presenting the various strategies that professional communities employ to deal with substitutes, we describe how turf challenges among health professions generally unfold. We use the term *claimant* to refer to the profession that presents itself as a substitute; the term *defender* refers to the profession being challenged with substitution.

The Nature of Substitutes

Substitutes exist for all health professions, though certainly not for all services of every profession. Table 4.1 gives examples of occupations and professions that can substitute for some or many of the tasks performed by the defender professions. Dental hygienists and dental lab technicians can perform some of the tasks of dentists, for instance, and in certain states or provinces of Canada, these professions legally can practice independently of dentists (Morganstein, 1989). (Dental lab technicians in the independent practice of denture construction and fitting commonly are referred to as denturists.) As another example, optometrists are a substitute for much of the work domain of ophthalmology (an MD specialty), as they have the legal right in most states to administer drugs as well as examine vision problems. Many optometrists support a movement to achieve the legal right to perform surgery as well, extending the breadth of the substitution challenge to ophthalmology. Not included in Table 4.1 are the many alternative healers, such as acupuncturists, herbalists, and naturopaths, who serve as additional substitutes for many of the professionals listed in the table.

Substitute occupations and professions may present themselves as complete or incomplete substitutes for a defender profession. The chiropractic profession provides a good example. It is possible for chiropractors to maintain "their claims to be able to treat all kinds of conditions and their theory that all illness is due to subluxations and that the only therapy is their removal" (Wardwell, 1982, p. 247). Adoption of this position essentially presents chiropractic as an alternative to mainstream medicine (MDs), based on an uncompromising view of its alternative knowledge base and the claimed capabilities of that base. In this case, the health profession has presented itself as a complete

Table 4.1. Substitutes for Selected Health Professions.

Profession	Substitute occupations and professions[a]
Administrators, health care	general business administrators and clinicians without health care administration entry education (P)
Administrators, long-term care	general business administrators and health care administrators without long-term care entry education (P)
Chiropractors	physical therapists (P), physicians (P)
Dental hygienists	dentists (P), dental assistants (S)
Dentists	dental assistants (S), dental hygienists (S), denturists (S), oral surgeons (S)
Denturists	dentists (P)
Dietitians	dietetic assistants (S), dietetic technicians (S)
Medical record administrators	noncredentialed personnel (P), medical record technicians (S)
Medical technologists	pathologists (P), medical lab technicians (S)
Nurse anesthetists	anesthesiologists (P)
Nurse-midwives	lay midwives (P), obstetricians (P)
Nurses, registered	physician assistants (P), physicians (P), licensed practical nurses (S), nurse assistants and aides (S), physical therapists (S), recreational therapists (S), respiratory therapists (S), other therapists and technicians (S)
Occupational therapists	occupational therapy assistants (S), physical therapists (S), recreational therapists (S), registered nurses (S), other therapists (S)
Optometrists	ophthalmologists (P), opticians (S), optometric technicians (S)
Pharmacists	physicians (P), pharmacy technicians (S)
Physical therapists	chiropractors (P), physicians (P), occupational therapists (S), physical therapy assistants (S), other therapists (S), registered nurses (S)
Physician assistants	nurse practitioners (P), physicians (P), registered nurses (S)
Physicians—DOs	MDs (P), others listed as substitutes for MDs
Physicians—MDs	DOs (P), chiropractors (S), dentists (S), nurse anesthetists (S), nurse-midwives (S), nurse practitioners (S), optometrists (S), physician assistants (S), podiatrists (S), psychologists (S), surgical assistants (S), various therapists and technologists (S)
Podiatrists	physicians (P), chiropractors (S)
Psychologists	medical social workers (P), psychiatric nurse practitioners (P), psychiatrists (P), other counselors (P)
Radiologic technologists	noncredentialed personnel (P), radiologists (P)
Recreational therapists	occupational therapists (S), other therapists (S), therapeutic recreational assistants (S)
Respiratory therapists	registered nurses (S), respiratory therapy technicians (S)
Social workers, medical	other counselors (P), social service assistants (S)
Speech-language pathologists and audiologists	noncredentialed personnel (P)

[a]P = substitutes for the *primary* work domain of the profession; S = substitutes for *secondary* tasks of the profession.

alternative to a mainstream health profession. Or the substitute health profession may limit its claim to a reduced set of tasks seen as appropriate to its distinctive knowledge base—as when chiropractic narrows the claims for its spinal manipulation therapy to *only* neuromusculo-skeletal conditions (Wardwell, 1982).

A particular kind of partial substitution occurs when one profession claims some of the more routine tasks of the other profession. The underlying dynamic involves a defender profession with a range of tasks, some of which require complex knowledge, others less complex knowledge. Typically this profession has become highly specialized. The claimant profession argues that minute specialization is unnecessary for the defender profession's more routine tasks. Indeed, the routine nature of the tasks often means that the requisite knowledge is not complex, making it easier to transmit and thus more accessible to another profession. The distinctiveness of the claimant profession in this case is the narrow range of tasks it would like to perform.

The search for vulnerable, routinized tasks by a claimant profession is a *task probe* strategy. Essentially the claimant is searching for potential weaknesses in a defender profession. Generally, there are two "task zones" that can be identified by such a search: abandoned zones and retentive zones. In the first case, a specialty profession may vacate a task area, creating an "abandoned zone." Optometry appears to have gained vision training as a task because the more specialized profession, ophthalmology, has no real interest in the function. Finding such a zone is advantageous for all parties because interprofessional conflict can be minimized. Typically, however, task zones are "retentive"—that is, the defender profession retains an active interest in the tasks, and will therefore oppose any challenges from claimants or will attempt to control the claimant profession. This condition is exemplified by dentistry's efforts to control dental hygienists and denturists.

Apart from routinization, claimant professions can also take advantage of other inadequacies of specialized professions in order to establish themselves as substitutes. For example, scientific medicine increasingly is criticized for its impersonal, bureaucratic style of practice (Maykovich, 1980; Wallis, 1991). Medicine also has emphasized "pill and scalpel" approaches that have worked well for acute disease but are less effective for the maintenance of health or for dealing with the chronic health problems that arise from aging and life-style. Nurse practitioners and certain health professions with an unorthodox knowledge base, such as holistic practitioners, strengthen their case as substitutes by exploiting the inadequacies of highly specialized, scientific medicine (Glazer, 1992; Frohock, 1992). Indeed, a recent analysis indicates that "unconventional medicine" is more frequently used in the United States than had been previously thought (Eisenberg, 1993).

Preventing the Challenges

Health professions have striven to prevent or minimize challenges from substitutes through use of legal strategies and through development of their knowledge base. Here we consider the primary strategies.

Legal Monopolization of a Work Domain

Health professions in the United States can establish a monopoly over substantive tasks or techniques through state licensure laws, as discussed in Chapter Three. This strategy can result in the prohibition of substitutes, as a legal statute may authorize only one health profession to provide the range of stipulated tasks and techniques. While no health profession has achieved a complete monopoly over its work domain, medicine and dentistry have been able to legally exclude substitutes from performing many tasks. And physicians, with their "unlimited licensure," are theoretically a substitute challenge to most other health professions. In Virginia, for example, medicine is legally defined as "the prevention, diagnosis and treatment of human physical or mental ailments, conditions, diseases, pain or infirmities by any means or method"—in other words, a virtually unlimited work domain (Code of Virginia 1950, 7A, Chap. 29, sec. 54.1-2900).

Legal Marginalization of Substitutes

The absence of a perfect monopoly for medicine and dentistry suggests a related strategy that the dominant health professions have pursued: legal marginalization of potential substitutes. Legal marginalization limits the extent of substantive task and technique overlap between a health profession and potential substitutes. Ideally for the dominant profession, the area of overlap contains tasks that are not core functions, thereby limiting a substitute's competitive impact to relatively unimportant areas. Not only is the substitute's competitive threat to specific tasks reduced, but the substitute's overall legitimacy and attractiveness to new recruits are diminished due to its restricted work domain. Unable to prevent the licensure of such health professions as optometry, chiropractic, and podiatry, for example, medicine essentially adopted a strategy whereby it attempted to marginalize, or limit, the tasks these substitutes can perform.

As marginalization is the more realistic strategy from the perspective of a health profession's *total* practice domain, it is important to note an additional aspect of this strategy. Marginalization implies encroachment on a profession's practice domain, but encroachment is not necessarily objectionable to the defender profession. Encroachment may be accepted by the defender profession or it may be contested. A profession may acquiesce in the encroachment because there is a need, such as pressure to increase productivity, for the substitute's services. Acquiescence, which commonly takes the form of a negotiated agreement between the professions concerning the substantive terms of the licensure law, enables the defender profession to control the extent of the overlap. The overlap is seen as marginal *and* in the interest of the acquiescing profession, conditions that free it of political conflict. Medicine frequently has adopted this approach in response to new technologies that physicians want to control, but do not directly utilize themselves. Of course, the profession that has accepted medicine's legal terms may later become more independent and seek a definition of its licensure code that medicine may find objectionable, as is the case with physical therapy. In this sense, then, acquiescence may serve as a foothold for a new profession to overcome the initial barrier of gaining licensure.

When encroachment is contested — two health professions cannot agree on the definition of each other's work domains — the implication is that the claimant profession does not accept the defender's view of an acceptable overlap of practice domains. The result is a political conflict over the encroaching profession's licensure code, a situation in which conflicting views over the sufficiency of education and training, as well as the resources of interest groups, determine the outcome of the fight. These battles occur frequently between medicine and health professions that have developed, or are attempting to develop, an independent client base (Begun and Lippincott, 1987). Medicine's conflicts with optometry, psychology, physical therapy, and chiropractic are examples of this dynamic.

New Knowledge Development

Whether a health profession is defending its own work domain or trying to encroach on other domains, a knowledge development strategy is important. This strategy requires that a profession develop the capacity to create knowledge that facilitates the performance of new tasks (or old tasks in new ways). As described in Chapters Three and Six, this capacity typically is institutionalized through a specialized subset of the professional community — academic researchers and teachers — and is an important strategy for creating legitimacy.

Development of knowledge is important for a specialized profession because it provides a defense mechanism. The continual development of new knowledge for the performance of tasks is a way to protect the profession's functional viability. Even though some tasks may become simplified and routine, newly developed complex knowledge assures that the profession will not ultimately be overtaken by routinization and hence greater accessibility to its knowledge base. The development of new knowledge provides a "protective dynamic" against ultimately being overtaken by a less specialized substitute.

The changing health care environment means that courts

and legislatures are less receptive to claims for legal monopoly and legal marginalization of substitutes. In fact, many stakeholders would be pleased to see more substitution possibilities in health care. As a result, health professions should rely less on legal strategies. The strategy of new knowledge development is an attractive alternative because it can involve satisfying key stakeholders' demands for meeting unmet needs or for more cost-effective treatments. For example, dentistry's response to dental hygiene's effort to legalize independent dental hygiene practice could include more intensive efforts to develop new tasks for dentistry, such as laser surgery, so that the profession could still retain market power while accommodating substitution for the dentist's more routine tasks.

Meeting Market Demands

Perhaps the best way for health professions to forestall the entry of substitutes into their work domain is to ensure that their services are cost-effective, accessible, and efficacious. To discourage the entry of competitors, monopolies should behave as they would in a competitive market. As market demands for health care buyers intensify, so too will pressures to allow more substitution possibilities among professions. To prevent this development, health professions can directly respond to the intensified market demands for cost-effectiveness and other stakeholder preferences.

Responding to the Challenges

If defender professions are unable to prevent challenges from substitutes, then they typically dispute the basic legitimacy of a substitute to perform certain tasks. Debate over the legitimacy of substitutes usually focuses on the adequacy of the substitute's knowledge base.

Scientific Basis

The scientific basis of the substitute profession frequently is a source of attack by the defender profession, particularly in the case of substitutes that are alternative healers. Orthodox health professions commonly have labeled alternative health professions as "quacks." The label is clearly intended to suggest that the unorthodox knowledge of the alternative profession does not result in competent performance of the tasks. The intention is to create a legitimacy problem directed at the very basis for the distinctiveness for the alternative profession — that is, its unorthodox knowledge base. The extreme claims made by some alternative health professions amplify their vulnerability. If chiropractic suggests that spinal manipulation really can cure pancreatic cancer, for example, the question of efficacy inevitably arises and the extreme claims provide the basis for the quack label. If such labeling is successfully implanted in the minds of buyers, mainstream professions will have taken a major step toward circumscribing the appeal of their unorthodox substitutes.

Claimant health professions, too, attempt to use labeling to attain legitimacy. Optometry and chiropractic, for example, both realizing the prestige derived from the title of "doctor," have fought political battles to gain access to the title. This issue becomes particularly contentious when an alternative health profession assimilates portions of orthodox knowledge. The expanded use of orthodox knowledge, despite the retention of some alternative knowledge and techniques, may appear to justify use of the "doctor" label. Of course, use of this label blurs the differences between the health professions — a decided advantage to the profession that formerly lacked access to the label.

Depth of Skills

Defender health professions usually can criticize the depth of the substitute's skills. This strategy derives from the basic fact that most substitute occupations and professions have been marginalized. Since they are limited in their work domain, they are vulnerable to the claim that the profession with the larger domain can perform a greater number of tasks. The implication is that the marginalized profession is therefore of less value. Mainstream medicine has often used this strategy against its chiropractic and osteopathic competitors.

Even when a substitute profession has not been marginalized, the depth of its skills can be challenged by a defender profession. Health care administrators question the ability of general business administrators to understand the distinctive management needs of health care organizations, for instance, while long-term-care administrators use the same argument relative to general health care administrators.

Insufficient Training

If the substitute's claimed tasks are in the "retentive" zone of the defender profession, it is common for the defender to pose a counterclaim of insufficient training: has the claimant really acquired adequate knowledge to perform the tasks? This strategy is not the same as the labeling strategy, which relates the charge of quackery to the unorthodox character of the knowledge. In this case, the knowledge is conventional — hence the counterclaim is that the knowledge is complex and therefore not readily accessible. The implication is that the claimant has not acquired *enough* knowledge to perform the tasks. It is also possible to link a "quality of care" dimension to the incompetency charge by arguing that the inadequate training will put consumers at risk — a claim that can be used to blunt the common argument that the claimant profession can perform the tasks more cheaply.

Collateralism

A truly powerful rebuttal by a defender profession typically builds on the challenge to the defender's training sufficiency. Often the first step is the collateralism argument. Rather than focusing only on the claimant's competency to perform the specific tasks, the emphasis is placed on the possibility that in performing these tasks, problems may arise for which the claimant profession is untrained. Dentistry, for instance, uses this argument against dental hygiene's effort to achieve independent practice for certain services. Inherent in the collateralism approach are several added dimensions. Since consumers are in prospective danger if the claimant is permitted to perform the tasks, such performance should require prior approval from the profession with superior training (usually physicians). This maneuver is essentially a fallback position. If the defender profession is in danger of losing monopoly over the tasks, it tries to establish positional control over the claimant. If a requirement of the defender's prior approval is not achieved, then the defender can argue that the claimant will at least require backup from the defender profession. Since backup suggests shared responsibility, especially with respect to malpractice, this again increases the justification for some kind of defender control over the claimant.

Indetermination

Another common response by the defender profession is to stress the indetermination inherent in the application of its knowledge base. In other words, competent performance of the claimed tasks entails "tacit" qualities of a practitioner that are acquired only through years of rigorous education and training. Members of the defender profession develop an intuition about certain task dilemmas and how to handle them. This quality arises only after years of training and experience, usually acquired under the guidance of an older, experienced practitioner. This argument is used in an effort to counter the notion that the claimant profession really can acquire competence through didactic education alone. Instead, competence requires the totality of the education, training, and experience that is involved in expertise. The indetermination argument often is used by a specialized profession because the claimant is held to be disadvantaged owing to its lack of specialization. Superiority is claimed to inhere in the very act of becoming a specialist.

Joint Demand

Finally, there is the joint demand rationale (Child and Fulk, 1982). This strategy builds on the indetermination argument by emphasizing that even if a task is relatively simple and routine, it is important for clients to have the reassurance of the superior professional judgment of the specialized profession. The argument focuses on assuaging the client's uncertainty. It can be used to combat not just claimant professions but also the growing commercialization of certain health care services (for example, weight reduction) and substitution of self-care for a profession's services.

Cost-Effective Knowledge

As described in the previous chapter, the bases for legitimacy of the health professions are shifting. Defending against substitute challenges by questioning the scientific basis of substitutes or through undocumented claims about indeterminism of the service is less and less likely to hold sway in the administrative, judicial, legislative, and regulatory arenas where substitute disputes are resolved. This means that health professions increasingly will need to rely on empirical evidence about the cost-effectiveness, efficacy, and accessibility of their services relative to substitutes. The comparative cost-effectiveness with which the profession and its substitute produce services has become a prominent dimension in the eyes of buyers in today's cost-conscious health care environment. The marketplace increasingly assesses a profession's cost-effectiveness relative to substitutes. A favorable differential yields a marketplace advantage over more costly but less effective substitutes. This advantage is particularly important for health professions that can provide services in new delivery systems (HMOs, PPOs) that emphasize cost-effectiveness.

With respect to cost-effectiveness, it is essential to recognize a nuance. As defender professions are well aware of the emphasis on cost differentials, relatively costly professions can try to close the gap by increasing the substitute's costs. For example, Feldstein (1988b) reports that registered nurses have supported pay policies that equalize the salaries of licensed practical nurses (LPNs) with their salaries. This increases the cost of the lower-priced LPNs, thereby eliminating their efficiency advantage as a substitute.

If the evidence is on the side of the claimant, the defender profession might be wise to negotiate a settlement that allows the claimant to offer the disputed service. While sacrificing some market power in the short term, the strategy of negotiating will meet the needs of powerful stakeholders and further the strategic adaptation of the defender profession. Numerous examples of this strategy are likely to be played out in managed care settings, as administrators of managed care plans negotiate for cost-effective services coordinated among several different health professions.

Other Strategies

Apart from strategies that emphasize a profession's knowledge and ability to perform tasks competently, health professions have used several other responses to challenges from substitutes. Each of them highlights relationships in the task environment that can facilitate or hinder a health profession's market power relative to substitutes.

Blocking Resources from Suppliers and Buyers

Members of a claimant profession may assert that they possess the competence to perform certain tasks, but competence alone may not be sufficient: material and financial resources also are crucial to the claimant's ability to perform the tasks. A defender profession can seek to prevent a substitute's access to important resources of suppliers and buyers.

Supplies of the material resources needed by a health profession to perform its work may be interdicted. As we shall see in Chapter Five, these resources can range from research and educational subsidies to hospital privileges to malpractice insurance. Educational subsidies provide support for growth in the profession. Research money contributes to the knowledge development that maintains the profession's competitiveness in skills. Hospital privileges provide access to equipment, labs, and domicile facilities, resources that frequently are crucial to a health profession's ability to perform everyday tasks. And access to malpractice insurance often determines whether practitioners can indeed perform a task.

A defender health profession can evaluate its substitutes' key resource needs and determine whether it is possible to limit the availability of resources. Since generally a defender profession already possesses the resources, it is advantaged in a competitive situation. As described earlier, medicine has used its control over hospital privileges to handicap competitors either through outright exclusion from the hospital or through limitations placed on the types of privileges. Medicine's control of federal research money through domination of the peer review process has advantaged it relative to substitutes. But the expense of specialized medicine — and the alleged lack of a correlation between expensive medical investments and health status — may provide a strategic opening for less specialized, "caring" health professions to claim a greater share of the research money than in the past. If so, their competitiveness as substitutes may be enhanced.

A critical resource is the knowledge base and training necessary to prepare for performing a task. Therefore, a defender profession may attempt to block a substitute's access to "legitimate" teachers. In a democratic society, it is virtually impossible for one profession to block another profession's access to knowledge in formal outlets such as journals and books. Blocking access to instruction by teachers has proved more feasible, however, and the defender profession may maintain that such a posture is appropriate given the alleged quackery of the claimant profession. Allopathic medicine often has used this strategy in its battles with chiropractic, optometry, and osteopathy. Of course, the defender health profession is well aware that education of outsiders by teachers from within the profession would contribute to the legitimation of the encroaching profession's claims to competence.

In the same way, a substitute's access to key buyers may be hindered by a defender profession. There are a variety of ways in which a substitute can be weakened. A claimant has a major problem if its services are not covered by insurance, for example, while its competitors are covered. Other sources of disadvantage include defining adverse conditions for reimbursement (for example, requiring the presence of a physician during performance of a task or requiring a physician's signature on the reimbursement form), providing lower reimbursement than is received by the defender profession, and requiring that the payment for a substitute's services be made through the defender profession. Feldstein (1988b) argues that the third factor — defining the defender as recipient of the payment — is the key for transforming a substitute into a "controllable," complementary health profession. This has been a key issue in the substitute conflict between nurse anesthetists and anesthesiologists.

For reasons argued previously, it is likely that strategies relying on the blocking of resources to substitutes will be less and less useful for the health professions. If not based on empirical evidence relating to cost-effectiveness and efficacy, such efforts are likely to result in charges of self-interested restraint of competition by the defender profession and thus to an amplification of pressure for government intervention.

Selective Assimilation

Another strategy frequently employed by defenders to deal with substitute occupations and professions is selective assimilation of the substitute's knowledge base and techniques. This strategy is always possible if a substitute's knowledge base does indeed generate an efficacious technique.

Unlike the previous set of stategies, this one is likely to become more common in the future because it increases the overall degree of substitute possibilities in the health care system — an outcome strongly demanded by stakeholders. An example is reflected in the work of a special NIH panel that has been established "to glean from nutritional therapy, touch therapy, acupuncture, naturopathy, homeopathy, herbal medicine and other alternative modes of healing a list of treatments that may be promising and can be tested in conventional experiments" (Brown, 1992, p. 8).

Relational Strategies

Relationships among substitute professions take place in the context of formal and informal role relations. Three important aspects of role relations influence substitute relationships. First, laws sometimes mandate hierarchical relationships between health professions. Second, health care is increasingly delivered in large-scale organizations, not in solo practices. As a result, much of the struggle for control over work occurs in an organizational setting, compelling health professions to position themselves advantageously in such settings. Third, client referrals can play a key part in defining role relations between professions.

A profession can seek to legally subordinate a potential substitute in order to prevent it from functioning independently. By legally requiring that the substitute function under the supervision of its competitor, the substitute's positional dependence is established. Sanctioned dependence essentially transforms the substitute into a structural complement of its competitor. Examples of this strategy are the requirements that the work of dental hygienists be supervised by a dentist and the work of physician assistants by a physician. It is the policy of the American Medical Association that allied health personnel should be under the supervision of practicing physicians (American Medical Association, 1990b, p. 31).

The laws, however, can be made much more complex than simple requirements of supervision. They can involve such details as empowering licensing boards to make case-by-case approval of requests from practitioners to use such subordinates. The power might even be extended to mandating prior approval of the specific tasks to be performed. This scrupulous attention to detail not only establishes the hierarchical subordination of the substitute, but it also discourages members of the dominant profession from using substitutes to increase the productivity of their practices. Hierarchical ordering by legal means is a strategy often acceptable to the subordinate profession, because it establishes its formal legitimacy.

With the growth of large-scale health delivery systems, role relations within organizations have become very important. Abbott (1988) indicates that it is not uncommon for an occupation in an organization to perform tasks that are formally reserved for another occupation. This informal division of labor essentially creates a de facto substitute; indeed, performance of the task constitutes a beachhead for a substitute to claim that task.

While the sharing of tasks might be convenient for a defender profession, it may be legitimating a substitute if informal performance leads to *formal* claims on the tasks. Further, more is at stake than legitimation of a substitute's task claim; allowing performance of the task may make an important contribution to a substitute's creation of its identity as a profession. Actual performance without formal recognition can create a solidifying sense of grievance among members of the substitute profession.

The context of employment is a variable that affects a profession's ability to maintain control over tasks (Child and Fulk, 1982). The emergence of large-scale delivery structures, in which routine tasks are objects of efficiency, provides an organizational opening for substitutes to gain control over routinized tasks. Conversely, these formal organizations are a source of challenge to specialized health professions.

If formal organizations are an emerging arena for substitute health professions, then a major focus of the substitution fights will likely be over the work process. Cook, Moris, and Kinne (1982) have argued that a crucial dimension of the work process is the relationships that are institutionalized among substitute health professions within the organizations. Different exchange relationships influence the extent to which potential substitutes control different tasks. For example, physicians may be tempted to use their gatekeeper role in managed care plans as a basis for undermining competitors. While such behavior risks being overridden by efficiency-minded administrators of the managed care plans, it is clear that control over the work patterns in formal health care organizations is an increasingly important strategic consideration in the competition between substitute health professions.

A more subtle dimension — the symbolic order — represents another important aspect of substitution conflict within formal organizations. Abbott (1988) points out that symbols of authority (such as titles and uniforms), as well as the use of exclusionary and coercive behavior, maintain a hierarchical division between different occupations. An elaborate culture of subordination is an important adjunct in the process whereby one profession attempts to control another. A potential substitute must contend with a symbolic order that continually defines it as "inferior" to its competitor — a condition that reinforces legal and formal subordination.

While large-scale health care organizations have become increasingly important, interprofessional relations with regard to clients remain a source of leverage in shaping substitute relationships. Such relationships can take a variety of forms: direct referral, consultation, and backup. If a health profession adopts a zero-sum view of its relationship with a substitute, as many have done in the past, its strategy is clear. It would deny the substitute profession patients and support for their care by withholding possible referrals, spurning a backup role, and accepting only a consultant role that provides an occasion for stealing the client. As a result, the substitute gains absolutely no support in its effort to maintain its client base.

Licensing laws sometimes create structural advantages and disadvantages in interprofessional relationships. Relative to psychiatry, for example, psychology has a more restricted work domain. If a patient needs drug therapy or surgery, psychologists must refer the patient to a physician. The laws configure referrals to the advantage of medicine — especially since the referral provides an opportunity to steal the patient, an action that apparently can be legitimated by the greater task range of physicians.

Another important intersection of law and client relationships concerns the definition of "primary care" status. Optometry has recently been successful in gaining the right to use drugs under state practice laws. Since the use of pharmaceuticals contributes significantly to the diagnostic capability of optometry, the legal change was important in its efforts to claim a "primary care" status in the provision of ophthalmic services. Of course, a successful claim to this status provides the profession with a weapon to subordinate its more specialized substitute in referral relationships.

While control over clients is a significant aspect of interprofessional relationships, other relations warrant mention. Denying substitutes membership in a profession's organizations, rejecting interprofessional forums, and refusing to teach substitutes are other forms of interprofessional relations that have been utilized by dominant professions to forestall substitution.

In the future, relational strategies are likely to move in the direction of cooperation rather than competition. As buyers push to reduce the cost of care through coordination of interdependent services, legal constraints on interprofessional relations will be viewed as barriers to more cost-effective, coordinated care. Many services can be delivered more cost-effectively by coordinated teams of professionals rather than individual providers (Richardson, 1991). Managed care systems rely on more extensive integration across professional boundaries. Professions will be asked to work in teams with substitutes, especially where the supply of certain professionals is limited. Arguments for hierarchical control traditionally have been based on quality issues — as, for example, in the case of the American Medical Association's position on supervision of physician assistants (American Medical Association, 1990b, pp. 229–230). These arguments will need to be supplemented by evidence showing that the arrangements are cost-effective and efficacious for consumers and do not inhibit access to care.

For similar reasons, professions will need to accommodate demands for cross-training of personnel, especially in settings where the supply of personnel cannot meet the demand. Alliances with substitute professions to create cross-training programs for selected markets would address a major concern of important buyer groups, such as small hospitals (Vaughan, Fottler, Bamberg, and Blayney, 1991).

Market Segmentation

There is a final strategy that can be used to define relationships between a health profession and its substitutes: the professions can develop different client niches. Most of the strategies examined thus far involve direct competition, where the focus typically has been to limit, hamper, and possibly prevent the existence of a substitute. Market segmentation, on the other hand, often becomes the means by which a health profession and its substitutes can establish an accommodation. This strategy acknowledges that the substitutes are going to exist. Appealing to different kinds of clients becomes a way to coexist.

The income of clients is a major basis for dividing the market, particularly when the competition occurs between a specialized health profession and less specialized substitutes. Optometry and ophthalmology, for example, have settled into a state of affairs in which the former more often serves lower-income clients and the latter higher-income ones. To appeal to a market segment, the substitute profession usually offers services at a lower price than the defender. While such accommodations often are relatively amicable, there is no guarantee that a health profession will continue to accept the accommodation. Such a reaction is demonstrated by the American Dental Association's call for programs to supply low-income people with low-cost dentures, a project designed to undermine their denturist substitutes (Feldstein, 1988a, pp. 494–495).

The underservice of inner city and rural areas by health personnel suggests that the geographic location of clients is another important dimension for client niches. If physicians are unwilling to locate in rural and inner city areas, this provides a possible niche for nurse practitioners. The niche may have unattractive features, of course, a condition that explains its existence. But exploitation of such an opening can be used to develop a beachhead for possible expansion into other locales, particularly after the demonstration of competence. On the other hand, a defender health profession, well aware of this dynamic, may oppose an accommodation with a substitute based on geography.

Another way for health professions to divide clients is on the basis of their health problems. Different professions can attempt to match their particular knowledge to the different problems of clients. As a result, conflicts based upon claims about quackery and educational sufficiency tend to be muted. Abbott (1988, p. 73) reports that different professions in the marital counseling area have reached such an accommodation.

A related basis for market segmentation is reflected in specialty niches. Highly specialized training of practitioners, as well as professional recognition of such training (for example, certification), increases the division of labor of health care tasks. As different types of practitioners are needed in order to perform tasks, substitutability among practitioners declines. As a result, *intra*professional competition decreases, and attendant "quality" claims of specialization blunt *inter*professional competition.

Compared to the standard strategies for dealing with substitutes, dividing markets according to specialized knowledge is particularly attractive. Other strategies have been criticized for their monopolistic character, which might invite antitrust initiatives or deregulation. Since specialized knowledge is seen as a source of progress, it is viewed more favorably and invites less critical attention. Market divisions can be justified as a natural by-product of progress. Specialization, however, requires a large and complex knowledge base.

Finally, the connection between client problems and particular organizations warrants emphasis. Clients with specific problems commonly are cared for in specialized institutions — another basis for development of a niche. The growing number of elderly, for example, provides an organizational niche not only for health professions in traditional nursing homes but also emergent institutional forms such as retirement communities. A health profession such as geriatric social work or gerontological nursing could develop a client base by gaining control of tasks in these institutions. Long-term-care administrators have successfully developed a specialty niche that is largely independent of health care administration. Moreover, client needs in other institutions may provide a niche for a health profession — the consultative needs of the courts, for example, have provided a supply of clients for psychologists and psychiatrists.

Conventional and Contemporary Strategies

To remain strong in the marketplace, health professions must manage their relationships with actual and potential substitutes. The conventional and contemporary strategies suggested for health professions to manage substitute relationships are listed in Table 4.2.

Historically, health professions have relied heavily on legal strategies to prevent the possibility of substitution. Stakeholders

Table 4.2. Strategies for
Managing Relationships with Substitute Professions.

Conventional Strategies

- Legally monopolize a work domain, and legally marginalize substitutes.
- Dispute the legitimacy of substitutes on grounds of quality.
- Block resource flows to the substitute from suppliers and buyers.
- Segment the market.
- Legally restrict the substitute's direct access to clients.
- In organizational settings, maintain hierarchical control over substitutes.

Contemporary Strategies

- Diversify the work domain through development of new knowledge.
- Respond to market demands for cost-effective, efficacious, accessible services, forestalling the need for substitutes.
- Dispute the legitimacy of substitutes on the basis of relative cost-effectiveness, accessibility, and efficacy.
- Selectively assimilate knowledge or tasks from substitutes.
- In organizational and managed care settings, form cooperative arrangements with substitutes.
- Directly compete with substitutes through expansion of the work domain.

---

in the judicial, legislative, and regulatory arenas are less likely to be receptive to such strategies in the future, however, suggesting that health professions should emphasize the development of new knowledge and ensure that their services are cost-effective, accessible, and efficacious to protect themselves from substitute challenges.

To deal with such challenges, health professions conventionally have disputed the legitimacy of substitutes on the grounds of quality, deprecating their scientific basis, depth of skills, and training while emphasizing the indetermination, collateralism, and joint demand inherent in the disputed service. Defender professions have sought to block resource flows from suppliers and buyers to substitutes and have refused to participate in the training of substitutes. They have created hierarchical subordination of substitutes in the workplace or insisted on interprofessional referral requirements.

Contemporary strategies for dealing with substitutes include the defender's selective assimilation of the knowledge base of substitutes. Also, substitute relationships are more and more likely to be shaped within large organizations, such as managed care companies, where management concerns for cost-effectiveness and other key stakeholder goals will constrain interprofessional relationships. While some degree of rivalry will remain inherent in relationships between professions and their substitutes, cooperative strategies for dealing with substitutes in the workplace are more likely to satisfy stakeholders' demands for greater cost-effectiveness, access, and efficacy in the health care sector. This means that more flexible, nonhierarchical relationships among substitutes will become increasingly common, as will more cooperative referral relationships.

We have generally considered the issue of substitute relationships from the standpoint of the defender profession. From the standpoint of claimant professions, we can expect greater encouragement of direct competition between substitutes from external stakeholders such as insurers, courts, and legislatures. While arrangements among substitutes in health care delivery organizations and managed care systems may be coordinated, greater competition among substitutes is likely outside those systems. There will be increased opportunities for claimant professions to challenge the defender's work domain through expansion of the claimant's domain. Recent successful examples of this strategy are the efforts of nurse practitioners to achieve prescriptive authority and those of physical therapists to achieve direct access to patients.

Apart from relationships with substitutes, professionals must strategically manage relationships with the buyers of their services and the suppliers of resources. In the next chapters, we explore the ways in which professions have handled these important market relationships.

Chapter Five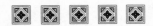

Managing Relationships with Suppliers

Most health professionals depend on a wide variety of suppliers in order to practice their profession. Suppliers to the professional community are the people and organizations that provide inputs — raw materials, human resources, technology, knowledge, space — used in the services performed by practitioners. Suppliers include both manufacturers and distributors of inputs to the professional community.

In one sense, teachers and researchers are suppliers, as well, because they "supply" practitioners with their knowledge base. But these exchanges are distinctive in that they occur long before the actual delivery of services by the professional, during the period of education and training. (Continuing education and the provision of new knowledge through journals and other outlets are exceptions.) The teaching and research inputs are so important that they generally are internalized by the professional community (Chapter Seven). In this chapter, we limit our discussion to relationships with suppliers outside the professional community.

Historically, the power of suppliers relative to health professionals has been constrained by distinctive features of the health care market — including the need to involve professionals,

112

third-party payers, and regulators in assessing the safety, efficacy, and availability of health care supplies. But as we shall
see, suppliers are gaining power in many areas, presenting new
challenges to the professions.

Types of Suppliers

One way to classify supplier relationships is by the type of supply. Equipment frequently is acquired by professionals or their
organizations to enable the practitioner to practice, as are space
and administration services. Malpractice insurance is a supply
required in many health professions. And in some professions,
suppliers are the source of products dispensed by practitioners.

Suppliers of Equipment

Many health professionals rely on equipment in order to deliver
their services. Equipment is costly for such specialties as radi-
ology in medicine, where a magnetic resonance imaging machine
can require a capital investment of $1 to $2 million. Radiologic
technologists and other imaging personnel also depend on that
equipment for the practice of their profession. Medical technologists use expensive, sophisticated equipment to analyze
blood and tissue. Respiratory therapists and physical therapists
may employ sophisticated and expensive machinery in their work
as well. Dentists use a range of equipment — from dental chairs
to instruments to imaging machines — and other independently
practicing professionals purchase a wide variety of equipment
for their offices.

For employed professions, the employing organization is
usually the supplier of equipment. Radiologic technologists work
with machines that are manufactured by private firms and marketed to hospitals and similar organizations. Automated systems for the storage of medical records are vended by private
manufacturers to hospitals, where the systems become part of
the technology applied by medical record administrators.

Organizations also may provide equipment for the delivery of services by nonemployees in order to attract their clientele,

as hospitals do for physicians. Traditionally hospitals have been labeled "the doctor's workshop" in recognition of this function. Beds, operating rooms, testing equipment, and more are provided to the many health professions that have treatment privileges within hospitals. These professions include MDs, DOs, optometrists, podiatrists, psychologists, dentists, chiropractors, nurse anesthetists, nurse-midwives, nurse practitioners, clinical nurse specialists, physician assistants, and others.

More and more health care services can be delivered outside the hospital setting. For example, radiologists and other medical specialists, such as ophthalmologists and urologists, increasingly are able to perform sophisticated surgeries outside the hospital. This change has forced many health professions to develop new supplier relationships in order to manage activities formerly administered by hospitals.

Suppliers of Products

In some cases, products are purchased from suppliers, altered or evaluated by the professional, and then dispensed to the client. These resources are unlike other supplies in that they are dispensed to clients. (The distinction between products and other supplies is problematic in the case of raw materials that become part of the client's body during the delivery of clinical services, such as tooth amalgam, artificial hips, and transfused blood.)

Typically, the products are purchased by professionals or their employing organization and then distributed in the course of their work. Physicians and pharmacists interact with suppliers of pharmaceuticals, as physicians prescribe and pharmacists dispense pharmaceuticals in the course of their work. Dentists form relationships with suppliers of dentures, orthodontia, tooth implants, and other products that are dispensed in the dental care delivery process. Optometrists dispense glasses and contact lenses purchased from lens manufacturers.

Other Suppliers

Other important supplies include personnel, space, malpractice insurance, and administrative services. Independently practicing professionals hire administrative and clinical staff and acquire space from real estate developers. Accounting services are a common example of administrative services purchased by health professionals. Malpractice insurance is a requirement for the delivery of services in many of the health professions, although its expense is onerous mainly for physicians in selected specialties.

As is the case with equipment, employing organizations mediate the relationship between employed professionals and suppliers of many of these inputs. Many professionals have been insulated from these relationships because suppliers have dealt with hospitals and other organizational entities, who in turn deal with the professionals on supply issues. As representatives of health care delivery organizations, health care administrators and long-term-care administrators frequently interact with supplier organizations and their representatives. As some clinical professions gain the ability to provide services independent of hospitals or other institutions, professionals are thrown into new relationships with suppliers. Physical therapists and psychiatric nurse practitioners, for example, who typically have depended on organizational employers, are opening independent offices.

The Structure of Supplier/Professional Relationships

Strategic challenges from suppliers generally come in two forms: one is the possibility of vertical integration, or entry into the professional service delivery market, by a supplier; the other is the exercise of economic power in the exchange between suppliers and members of the profession. Suppliers can exercise economic power more readily under certain conditions — when the suppliers are large, concentrated, and provide critical inputs, for example, and where there are few substitutes for the supplier's input. Under these conditions, suppliers can unfairly raise the prices of their inputs or threaten to disrupt services by withholding or delaying deliveries.

Suppose, for example, that the imaging manufacturing industry were monopolized by one firm that developed a more cost-effective but more complex imaging machine requiring extensive knowledge beyond that possessed by practicing professionals. The firm could argue that its own engineers and technicians should run the machine and interpret its output, rather than radiologists or radiologic technologists outside the firm. While such a situation is hypothetical, it illustrates the vulnerability that professions face when they use supplies that are developed outside the professional community. In fact, representatives of manufacturers frequently are involved in training professionals to use new technologies.

Professions have more control when suppliers are small in size, unconcentrated, and competitive with other suppliers. This ensures that suppliers cannot monopolize the market and raise prices and otherwise exert influence over individual professionals. A similar rationale motivates independently practicing professionals to seek multiple sites for admitting patients to hospitals: multiple sites reduce the professional's dependence on any one hospital.

Compared to other industries, direct challenges from suppliers are generally rare in the health industry due to the special nature of health services. Many supplies that are dispensed to consumers or used in the service delivery process are potentially harmful. As a result, a vast regulatory apparatus screens many of the medical devices and products before they are allowed in the market and then their utilization is monitored. Special restrictions accompany the use of many products, such as pharmaceuticals. The Food and Drug Administration, as well as the many sources of technology assessment mentioned in Chapter One, are involved in the assessment and monitoring process. Equipment and supplies are used in the educational process for new health professionals, giving educational institutions a voice in the screening and control of supplies, as well. The Academic Medical Centers Consortium is seriously involved in this activity.

Another sector that mediates relationships between suppliers and professionals is the third-party payer. Buyers of health services are concerned about the efficacy and cost of new equipment and products and are increasingly involved in screening assessment. A final constraint on the supplier's power is that suppliers frequently need the cooperation of professionals in order to develop new products and equipment. Suppliers are unable to assess the strengths and weaknesses of many products without the advice of knowledgeable health professionals who dispense or use the product.

Therefore, it often is in the interests of suppliers to work cooperatively, rather than competitively, with health professionals. (In fact, as we shall see, a danger for consumers is that health professionals may work too closely with certain suppliers and develop conflicts of interest.) All of these factors have insulated the health care professions from serious threats of entry or downstream integration by suppliers.

A special case of vertical integration occurs when one profession uses the services of another as a "supply." Most of the work of medical technologists is derived from physicians' orders, for instance. If the profession using the supply faces reduced demand in its own work domain, it may prefer to provide the service itself (vertically integrate) rather than use the supplier—particularly if the supplied service is lucrative, as some physicians have concluded is the case for laboratory work and dispensing of drugs. If competitive conditions are accentuated, conflict between professions with such supply relationships will intensify. As these conflicts sometimes escalate into defender versus substitute conflicts, they are discussed in more detail in the previous chapter.

In some professions, such as optometry, pharmacy, and ophthalmology, practitioners dispense products that are mass-produced by large and powerful corporations. Arguably the most prominent example of suppliers that have achieved significant power over a health profession is found in the case of the pharmaceutical industry and the pharmacy profession. The pharmaceutical industry not only controls the prices and quality of the product dispensed by pharmacists. It has, through its control over research and development and manufacturing techniques, diminished the profession's technical functions, leaving the profession essentially to perform more routine distributive functions. This has had the secondary effect of shifting the balance of power between the physician and the pharmacist.

By contributing less "value added" to the exchange, the pharmacist's clinical role has been reduced — thus weakening the position of the pharmacist relative to the physician in pharmacy's own struggle with medicine over control over the clinical aspects of drug therapy. Pharmacy now is attempting to redress this trend by emphasizing the pharmacist's education and role as drug therapy adviser and counselor, a strategy complicated by internal divisions between pharmacists educated under the old educational paradigm and those with newer educations.

New Challenges in Supplier/Professional Relationships

The triangular relationship between the pharmacist, pharmaceutical industry, and physician provides a good example of what may be an increasingly important challenge coming from the suppliers to health professionals. Many pharmaceuticals that formerly required a physician's prescription are becoming available directly to consumers — bypassing both pharmacists and physicians while increasing the power of manufacturers and distributors. Examples include drugs for the treatment of vaginal yeast infections, whose sale over the counter was approved by the FDA in 1990, sparking a $100 million marketing battle among manufacturers for shares of that market (Deveny, 1991). A similar development is the direct sale of eyeglasses and contact lenses to consumers armed with knowledge of their vision needs or who are willing to do trial-and-error shopping. The generic drug movement, stimulated largely by consumer groups and government, is an example of buyers working with suppliers to alter the service delivery of a health profession. With the explosion of technology in computing, lasers, genetic engineering, and the like, many suppliers could be in a position to alter the relative power of not only the health professions but other key stakeholders. By increasing their control over new product innovations, powerful suppliers also challenge the position of academic institutions, the traditional source of new knowledge and technology for the health professions. This is particularly true if the innovations make it possible to transform the otherwise "indeterminate" technologies controlled by the professions into more "technical" and systematized products that can be dispensed by lower-level personnel or even directly to consumers.

For professionals who depend on large organizations for employment or equipment and space, alliances between suppliers and employers are a particular challenge. To the extent that professionals are insulated from supplier relationships by their employers, the professionals lose control over the development of that relationship. Physicians have been quite successful at controlling hospitals' selection of medical supplies and equipment. But with rising cost-containment efforts, health care delivery organizations are becoming more rigorous in monitoring and influencing the purchase of supplies and equipment. Multihospital systems and hospital chains have developed highly structured guidelines for justifying equipment purchases, and consulting companies offer their own models to guide hospitals in these investments (M. Wagner, 1990).

In summary, then, challenges from suppliers, while historically constrained by the distinctive nature of health services, are expanding. The strategies that follow have helped professional communities manage their changing relationships with suppliers.

Managing Supplier Relationships

Professions develop strategies to reduce their dependence on suppliers or create stable and predictable relationships with them. When powerful suppliers exist outside the professional community, health professions have worked to create joint demand for both the supply and the profession's services. Moreover, professions have striven to minimize the threat of forward vertical integration by manufacturers and distributors into the work domain of the professional: the delivery of services.

Vertical Integration by Suppliers

Many health professions have created legal requirements that certain products be dispensed only by a credentialed professional.

If consumers want the product or the equipment, they must purchase the services of the professional as well. Demand for the equipment or product is linked with demand for the professional's service. This joint demand strategy forestalls the possibility of forward integration by the supplier into the retail sale of the product or the delivery of services using the equipment. Certain drugs can legally be prescribed only by physicians and selected practitioners, for example, and dispensed by pharmacists. This policy minimizes the threat that pharmaceutical manufacturers can sell directly to consumers or that employers of pharmacists can substitute clerical personnel (or robots) for pharmacists. In most jurisdictions, dentures can be dispensed only by dentists, a joint demand that denturists argue is unnecessary.

As is the case with other legal strategies, achieving legal authorization of joint demand requires that professions deal with regulators, policy makers, and the legal system. Professions with critical supplier relationships are quite involved in these influence-building activities — particularly because large supplier firms and their associations are engaged in similar activities.

The possibility of vertical integration by suppliers is a form of substitute challenge, since vertical integration by suppliers creates a new substitute for the profession's services. As a result, other strategies that health professions have pursued to reduce the threat of suppliers becoming substitutes are similar to those discussed in Chapter Four on substitute relationships. Challenging the legitimacy of a supplier's claims to be able to perform a task is a common strategy. Pharmacists and physicians have argued that direct sale of certain pharmaceuticals over the counter is dangerous to consumers owing to potential side-effects, drug interactions, or the danger of inappropriate application. Professions have questioned suppliers' ultimate incentives with regard to the health of consumers, arguing that suppliers are for-profit companies with different incentives than professionals.

Another common way to build joint demand is to emphasize the professional's role in judging or altering a supply (for example, a lens, drug, or denture) or interpreting the output of a piece of equipment (for example, an imaging machine or blood chemistry analyzer) during delivery of the professional service. If the products are not altered or judged or manipulated by the professional, they are subject to delivery by non-professionals. Home pregnancy tests, for example, require little or no professional judgment to perform or interpret, and now they are marketed directly to consumers. Building joint demand has involved the professions in underscoring the key role of professional judgment (indeterminate knowledge) and the shortcomings of trial-and-error, self-administered use of the product or equipment. The vision care professions have been accused of pressuring manufacturers to stop mail-order contact lens replacement services that do not include a personal fit of lenses on the premises — an example of the joint demand argument ("State Investigates . . . ," 1992).

The fact that the vision care professions are being investigated for antitrust violations in the example just cited reflects the new context for supplier/professional relationships. The professions can no longer claim to be insulated from profit-making incentives — and therefore so different from supplier business firms. Legal, legislative, and regulatory decisions about a supplier's entry into the direct delivery of care are more and more likely to be made on the basis of such values as cost-effectiveness, efficacy, and access. It is likely, too, that more supplies will be marketed directly to consumers — the expanding home care market is an example. This development is similar to routinization of the profession's knowledge base, discussed in previous chapters, in that it calls for greater investment by the profession in developing new knowledge in order to fight off the usurpation of parts of its work domain by suppliers.

Professions can anticipate future strategic challenges by keeping informed about developments in their supplier sector. For instance, professions must ensure that new knowledge about products and equipment is continually infused into their educational process, both initially and through continuing education. This gives more credence to the professions' position that they, not the supplier, should administer or dispense the supply. To monitor and shape the development of new equipment or product innovations in the interests of the profession, health professions can work to involve their members in the research and development of new supplies. Professions such as pharmacy have created educational tracks for members who are interested in such research.

Changes in the nature of key supplies can have interesting effects on interprofessional relationships. The diversity of sophisticated new imaging machines has meant that technologists (for example, sonographers and computed tomography technologists) have assumed more responsibility for interpreting results and dealing with manufacturers' representatives, giving technologists more power relative to radiologists (Barley, 1990). To the extent that a profession can quickly incorporate new knowledge about critical supplies into their educational processes, the profession is better prepared to adapt to new realities in role relations among professions.

Cooperative Linkages

Like most external linkages, cooperative relationships with suppliers can be used to create opportunities for professions. Links with important suppliers can be developed in order to advance joint goals. Historically, health professions have elicited financial resources and other support from major suppliers in exchange for publicity in the professional community or increased access to professionals. Pharmacists, for example, have benefited from the drug industry's support of their profession through contributions to professional associations, scholarship funds, and the like. Suppliers of imaging equipment have aided educational programs for radiologic technologists by donating equipment — thus addressing the joint goal of the profession and its suppliers to produce an adequate number of professionals (Appleby, 1990). Hospital suppliers like Abbott Laboratories support activities of the professional association of health administration educators. Pharmaceutical and supply firms have been generous in the benefits provided to physicians who might order their products.

In today's environment, such arrangements may be harmful to a profession's legitimacy in that supplier/professional relationships can be viewed as too cozy. Close relationships with suppliers could lessen the professional's objectivity in selecting the most appropriate supply. The promotional activities of pharmaceutical firms, such as giving gifts to physicians, as well as the objectivity of their advertisements in medical journals, have been criticized by the FDA, legislative committees, and other external stakeholders. To address this problem and reassure external stakeholders, professional communities must develop and enforce ethical standards about accepting the largess of suppliers.

Alternative Suppliers

As noted above, market conditions affect the ability of professions to avoid economic pressures from suppliers. Thus, professional communities can strive to create competitive conditions in their supplier industries through lobbying for appropriate legislation and other means. Physician groups have pressed for legislation that would foster greater competition in the malpractice insurance industry, for instance. Professional communities can encourage their members to experiment with different suppliers or to switch suppliers from time to time. This strategy also requires that professionals keep their "switching costs" to a minimum — that is, avoid heavy investment in one particular brand of equipment or product. Professionals should be wary of the extreme product differentiation that would allow suppliers to create monopoly conditions in the market for their particular supply. Common examples of such differentiation are new brand-name drugs that do not have accepted generic substitutes.

In an extreme situation, a profession might even consider backward integration — incorporation of the supply function within the professional community, in the way that professions have incorporated teachers and researchers within the community. While this option is unlikely for most supplies, there are exceptions. For instance, groups of professionals have created self-insurance pools for malpractice liability in response to conditions in the insurance industry. The movement of many physician and other services outside the hospital into ambulatory settings owned by professionals is a form of backward integration, as well, with professionals relying less on hospitals for space, equipment, admitting privileges, and other needs.

Of particular concern to external stakeholders are the cases where practitioners invest in or even own supplier firms, such as physician ownership of medical laboratory or imaging facilities. The evidence is overwhelming that such arrangements often result in a greater volume of the "supplies" being ordered (Rodwin, 1992). This raises questions about the practitioner's commitment to the health of the client versus the financial interest of the practitioner. In the aggregate, these situations seriously threaten the legitimacy of the profession. Thus professions are well advised to vigorously enforce conflict-of-interest norms regarding involvement in the supply function. The alternative to such a strategy is greater scrutiny by external stakeholders.

Countervailing Power

The professional who purchases supplies is relatively powerless in relationships with supplier firms, which are inevitably larger and more economically powerful than the individual. As Porter (1980, p. 27) points out: "Suppliers selling to more fragmented buyers will usually be able to exert considerable influence in prices, quality, and terms." Therefore, collective strategies within the professional community are required. Professionals in similar supplier relationships can form loose alliances (even across professions if the same large firm supplies different professions) or can use their associations to bargain with suppliers. Groups of professionals and associations then can realistically threaten to change suppliers or develop a new supply source. Organizations of professionals can hire staff to investigate the price and quality of suppliers and then communicate that information to members. This strategy reduces the information and shopping costs of individual practitioners and also promotes more competitive conditions in the supplier sector.

Conventional and Contemporary Strategies

In sum, then, professions can influence their relationships with suppliers even when those suppliers hold a great deal of power over the profession. Table 5.1 shows conventional and contemporary strategies for dealing with suppliers. Conventional strategies

Table 5.1. Strategies for Managing Relationships with Suppliers.

Conventional Strategies

- Legally require that only credentialed professionals dispense certain products and operate certain equipment.
- Challenge the legitimacy of direct market transactions between suppliers and buyers, underscoring the key role of professional judgment.
- Elicit resources from major supplier organizations in exchange for publicity within the profession, access to professionals, and the like.

Contemporary Strategies

- Accommodate the entry of suppliers into delivery of products directly to consumers when such arrangements result in more cost-effective, accessible, and efficacious services. Emphasize development of new knowledge to stay ahead of such changes.
- Support the creation of competitive conditions in key supplier sectors.
- Join fellow professionals or other professions in purchasing groups.
- Work with suppliers in developing new products.
- Prevent practitioners from forming relationships with suppliers that may exploit the consumer/professional relationship.

---

to deal with suppliers have emphasized keeping the suppliers from having direct access to clients. Contemporary strategies, on the other hand, recognize that such access is a response to stakeholders' demands and should be accommodated. Instead of opposing the entry of suppliers, professional communities can choose to emphasize the development of new knowledge, work to create competitive conditions in supplier industries, aggregate into collective organizations in order to bargain with suppliers, and bridge with suppliers in order to keep abreast of changes that will affect the profession's relationships with other professions, buyers, and key stakeholders. Finally, professions must act boldly to prevent their members from forming relationships with suppliers that exploit the client/professional relationship — thereby risking government intervention or further erosion of the profession's legitimacy.

Chapter Six ◈ ◈ ◈ ◈ ◈

Managing Relationships with Buyers

For health professionals, probably the most consequential changes in recent years have been revisions in the relationships between practicing professionals and the buyers of their services. Professionals face critical challenges in learning about, managing, and shaping these changes. Here we examine the strategies they can pursue to accomplish that learning, managing, and shaping.

Market Structure and Buyer/Professional Relationships

Buyers are those, both individuals and organizations, who purchase the services of a health professional in a market exchange. Buyers purchase these services through direct transactions or through the employment relationship. This category of stakeholders includes employers, individual consumers, and third-party payers.

In a professional service transaction, there is a direct provider/client relationship that involves compensation for the provision of services. The source of compensation may be directly from the consumer or from a third party that pays a share of the cost for the consumer. Third-party payers include private insurance companies such as Blue Shield and commercial companies, government programs such as Medicare and Medicaid, and certain HMO and PPO arrangements with providers. In contrast, an employment transaction stems from an employer/employee relationship wherein the health professional is compensated for services stipulated by the employer. The most obvious employment relationship in the health care industry is between various health professionals and hospitals, but this transaction would also include those hired by such organizations as home health agencies, HMOs, and physician's offices. Members of the same health profession may deal with different kinds of buyers. Income for nurses may come predominantly from an employment relationship with hospitals, but nurses are also employed by such organizations as nursing homes, physician's offices, and HMOs, and some of them practice independently.

For several health professions, clients are accessible only upon referral from other providers—their services are ancillary to another provider's or are only to be performed under the ultimate direction of another provider. For example, physical therapists and occupational therapists have been able to offer services only on referral from physicians. Referring professions can constrain the demand for a profession's services by withdrawing their recommendation. If the referring profession faces reduced demand in its own work domain, it may prefer to provide the service itself (vertically integrate) rather than referring. The same may be true if the referred task suddenly becomes lucrative, as some physicians have concluded is the case for laboratory work and dispensing of drugs. Dentists may do more teeth cleaning themselves if they face low demand for other dental work, thus lowering the demand for dental hygienists. Health professionals who depend heavily upon referrals, particularly from members of other health professions, must strategically manage their relationships with them. For this reason, many of the strategies outlined here for managing buyers also are relevant for dealing with referring professions.

The market in which buyer/professional transactions take place significantly affects the buyer/professional relation. We first inspect strategies directed at shaping the supply and demand for the services of a profession.

Supply Side of the Market

On the supply side of the market, the requirement of a license to practice is a formidable structural barrier for entry into a market. Only those sanctioned by law may perform the acts defined in the legislation, so those without a license are excluded as potential practitioners. Generally, health professions that have attained licensure have greater power to restrict the number of practitioners than professions without licensure. As discussed in Chapter Three, other forms of public credentialing, namely certification and registration, are less exclusionary because they allow uncertified and unregistered individuals to practice the profession. Professions often seek to expand the benefits of certification or registration, however, by seeking requirements that employers hire only certified or registered professionals. This strategy reduces the potential supply of professionals, thus increasing the bargaining power of credentialed professionals. Medical record administrators have pursued this strategy, as hospitals are required to hire or contract with a credentialed medical record administrator to meet accreditation standards.

The power of certification extends to specialty certification as well. Through specialty certification, the profession develops greater control over the supply of specialists of different types — thus increasing buyers' dependence on the professional community to supply an appropriate number. Nursing, with its new centralized control over specialty certification, hopes to gain the benefits of this strategy, although there are doubts that these benefits will be realized (Styles, 1982). Medicine has continued to expand the impact of its specialty certification system. Beginning in 1992, clinical medical department heads in hospitals must be board-certified in the clinical specialty of the department in order to meet JCAHO accreditation standards.

In addition to licensure, certification, and registration, there is another structural feature of the supply side of the market: the training and education of a profession's members. One credentialing strategy described in Chapter Three — standardized education and training under strong professional direction — has consequences for the supply of a profession's members. The medical profession provides a good example. Early in this century, the American Medical Association supported the inspection of medical schools by The Carnegie Foundation. The foundation's analysis, the Flexner Report, recommended improvements in medical education and was used to rationalize the closure of many medical schools. The report claimed that too many physicians were being produced: what medicine needed, it argued, was fewer and better-trained practitioners. With the ensuing passage of state practice laws requiring graduation from approved schools as a condition of licensure, as well as AMA's Council of Medical Education in control of the accreditation of medical schools, the medical profession was able to reduce the number of medical schools and thus the supply of practitioners.

The medical profession's control over medical education extends into the nature of the educational process itself. Educational requirements for entry into medical school, the size of classes, the length of training, and the nature of the courses also affect the supply of practitioners. Rigorous entry requirements, small class sizes, and lengthy training help to restrict supply and promote an increased rate of return on the medical education of current practitioners. Federal health manpower policies, which subsidized the expansion of medical education beginning in the 1960s, ultimately eased these supply restrictions. One consequence of increased supply can be lower relative incomes. Reinhardt (1985, p. 371) says that "the decline in the ratio of physician income to average employee compensation probably reflects the sustained rise in the physician-population ratio during the 1970s." Also the increased supply of physicians has contributed to a "buyer's market" for managed care plans (for example, HMOs and PPOs) that impose reimbursement limits on practitioners.

Many health professions have not attained a standardized training process under their firm control, however, and often the result is a more elastic supply of practitioners. Several allied health professions are in this situation. Their education often can be undertaken in community colleges, which have been promoted as attractive educational sites due to their responsiveness to local needs. The relative lack of task complexity means that the training period is shorter and less complicated.

A third structural feature of the supply side concerns potential substitutes for a health profession. Although this issue was examined extensively in Chapter Four, we must emphasize that substitutes effectively increase the supply of practitioners and the resulting rivalry reduces the market power of the profession compared to a market with no substitutes. A final structural feature of the supply side of the market concerns internal competition, a topic covered in Chapter Seven. Basically greater levels of internal competition in a profession reduce its market power relative to buyers.

For these reasons, health professions often have striven to control the quantity of new entrants through licensing and certification, standardized education, and discouraging substitution and internal competition. Today such restrictions are likely to invite intervention, however, requiring that professions devote greater efforts to monitoring and satisfying society's demands for services. Yet the health professions give surprisingly little attention to assuring an adequate supply of practitioners. Abbott (1988) has pointed out that several professions have lost control over work domains due to their inability to respond rapidly to increases in demand, citing psychiatry's loss of control over the domain of psychotherapy as one example. If powerful buyer groups are unable to secure adequate quantities of workers, they may decide to educate workers themselves — outside the professional community. Integrated health care systems have even pursued the goal of becoming "self-sufficient in the production of health personnel" (Brown and McCool, 1990, p. 88). Such developments frequently refer to occupations requiring shorter periods of formal education, such as nurse aides trained by nursing home chains or pharmacy technicians trained by retail pharmacy chains, but the threat is there for other professionals as well. In Chapter Seven, we return to the issue of managing the size of the profession.

Demand Side of the Market

Certain features of the demand side of the market have an important effect on buyer/professional relationships. In light of the importance of third-party reimbursement for health services, insurance coverage of a profession's services is a basic demand-side consideration. A health profession whose services are insured has an advantage over an uninsured profession because insurance has the effect of reducing the price of the insured profession's services. The result is higher demand for the insured profession. Health professions, recognizing this, have long lobbied for coverage of their services by third-party payers, though conflicts have emerged over direct reimbursement versus reimbursement through institutions or through another provider (often a physician). It is due to the implications for demand for their services that health professions are lobbying the Clinton administration for inclusion in any new national health insurance program.

Recent attention to the large number of Americans lacking health insurance raises an important issue. Health insurance subsidies for low-income people are particularly attractive to health professions because subsidies increase demand for care (Feldstein, 1988a). Without the subsidy, some people would be unable to pay and are thus effectively removed as a factor in the marketplace. As noted by Kosterlitz (1991, p. 1569), "doctors and hospitals, because they want everyone to be able to afford their services, are concerned that at least 33 million Americans lack health insurance."

In evaluating the effects of insurance on the demand for a health profession, it is important to remember that its impact extends beyond direct coverage of a profession's specific services. Under Medicare's original cost-plus formula for reimbursing *hospitals*, for example, a large proportion of nursing wages could be passed on to the federal government. Demand for nurses increased and, simultaneously, demand became more inelastic with regard to wages. While this situation was advantageous for nurses, the diagnosis-related grouping (DRG) reimbursement process under Medicare—with fixed reimbursement for each patient based on diagnosis—has negative demand implications for nurses. Since personnel represent such a high proportion of hospital costs, hospitals may now have an incentive to reduce the number of nurses and their wages in order to bring costs within DRG rates.

While examination of the demand side of the market typically focuses on insurance, other recent developments have important consequences for health care professions. With the de-emphasis on hospitals as comprehensive centers of care due to their high cost, a process of institutional decentralization has developed. Ambulatory surgery centers, freestanding primary care centers, specialized facilities (birthing, cardiac rehabilitation, and imaging centers) and home health agencies are becoming more prominent. HMOs have increased in quantity and so too have the number and scale of physician group practices. With an increasingly aging population, nursing homes will assume greater institutional prominence in the health care system. This decentralization and fragmentation of the health system should increase the number and diversity of buyers who demand the services of various health professions. This development is especially likely to benefit nurses and allied health practitioners as these new delivery organizations attempt to optimize their productivity.

Changes in population demography and illness patterns affect the demand for services of the different professions, as described in Chapter One. The opportunities for health professions to meet growing demands for chronic illness care — and to tailor their services to specific groups, such as women, racial and ethnic minorities, and the elderly — are legion. Professional associations can support this matching of buyer demand with professional services by monitoring demographic and illness patterns and promoting educational programs to train practitioners in meeting new demands.

Finally, in Chapter Four we mentioned the range of tasks a profession performs within its work domain. Generally, the wider the work domain, the greater the profession's economic value. Demand for its members should increase, which in turn increases market power. This is the major reason why nurses have attempted to gain the legal right to perform a greater number of tasks. As delineated in Chapter Four, stakeholders' pressure for greater substitution is likely to grow, making expansion of the work domain a strategy of continuing viability.

Strategies for Managing Relationships with Buyers

In this section, the analysis shifts from the market context of the buyer/professional exchange to an examination of strategies that can be used by health professions to manage direct relationships with buyers. As was the case with substitute and supplier relationships, historically the professions have relied on legal strategies and appeals to legitimacy in order to maintain significant power over the buyer sector.

Legal Restrictions on Buyer Power

Health professions have used the force of law to define advantageous relationships with buyers. Essentially, this occurs either by constraining the actions of a buyer that have unfavorable consequences for a health profession or by compelling actions that have favorable consequences. Many health professions have inhibited the employment of professionals by nonprofessionally owned corporations through laws and regulations, for instance, and have restricted the dissemination of price and quality information that would allow buyers to shop around more easily.

The medical profession's long battle over managed care is exemplary of the legal strategy. Earlier in this century organized medicine obtained Blue Shield enabling laws that constrained the activity of HMOs, and efforts were made to eliminate HMOs altogether based on the argument that they violate laws against the corporate practice of medicine (Kissam, 1978). These historic efforts have a current form. Physicians lobbying state legislatures have sought laws that reportedly "would be very costly, if not ruinous, to managed care plans, especially PPOs" (Crenshaw, 1991, p. H4). Legislative proposals designed to inhibit managed care include requirements by PPO networks to admit "any willing provider," prohibitions against "gatekeeper" physicians (whose referral to specialists is required for specialists' services to be reimbursed), and restriction of utilization review, benefit design, and benefit differentials (Cooper and Green, 1991).

The initiation of lawsuits is another form of legal strategy. Litigation involving managed care plans has the possibility of including insurers and company sponsors as liable parties in suits initiated by patients over care (Crenshaw, 1991). Currently physicians and other clinical professionals are the liable parties, and presumably it is in their interest to support a broadening of the scope of liability since it would weaken managed care by making insurers vulnerable to patient's lawsuits. In a different legal arena, a variety of activities by physicians and other providers have been scrutinized by the federal government for possible violations of antitrust law by professionals (Greenberg, 1991). But antitrust litigation on behalf of professionals may be possible in the future if buyers were to develop and use significant monopsonistic power.

Challenges to the Legitimacy of Buyer Power

Chapter Three examined the importance of legitimacy to health professions if they are to establish their viability in the market. Without social acceptance, a clinical health profession is unable to develop a patient base, a prerequisite for survival. Using a legitimacy strategy against buyers is often an outgrowth of the profession's position that the provider/patient relationship is the basis for the actual health service — any external payer is viewed as an outsider. By raising issues about alleged interference in the service relationship by outside parties, clinical health professions attempt to gain public and political support to pressure the parties.

Actions by the medical profession exemplify use of the legitimacy strategy. The profession's historic attacks on the federal government's involvement in paying for health care as "socialized medicine" were an effort to constrain the federal government's role as a buyer. When the role finally emerged in the form of Medicare, the usual, customary, and reasonable (UCR) reimbursement process gave physicians great market freedom in their service pricing. Appeals to "free markets" and concern about government intrusion into economic life are strongly held values in the American political culture. Until the growth of Medicare spending and the nation's deficit prompted development of the RBRVS reimbursement process, these values were used to rationalize a very favorable payment system for physicians.

A current expression of the legitimacy strategy involves managed care. Physicians Who Care, an association opposed to HMOs, has attempted to persuade the public that HMOs offer inferior medical care. One spokesperson for the organization has claimed that "senior citizens are being herded into HMOs by the federal governments to save money" and that "they are losing their medical rights and their freedom to choose their own doctor" (Rundle, 1987, p. 1). Dr. David V. Himmelstein, an organizer of Physicians for a National Health Plan, contends that a prominent proposal for reorganizing the health delivery system using HMOs — the Enthoven Plan — would cause "severe restriction of patient choice" and physicians would be employees of a "profit-making company whose main interest is in its bottom line and is free to dictate clinical decision-making" (Abramowitz, 1992, p. H7). While these critics of managed care espouse different philosophies, the rhetoric of "medical rights," "freedom to choose," "profit making," and "dictation" of clinical decision making is an attempt to damage the credibility of managed care buyers. Essentially, these buyers are viewed as threatening important values in the provider/patient relationship, a relationship that polling suggests is a sensitive one for the public (Toner, 1993). The implication of a successful attack along these lines is clear: that consumers should withdraw their support in order to protect themselves.

Legitimacy bears directly on physician reimbursement in managed care programs. The financial viability of these programs depends on minimizing utilization rates and treatment costs. Moreover, physician reimbursement is related to limiting treatment costs. A General Accounting Office analysis of payment incentives offered to physicians by HMOs stated: "If not properly controlled, such incentives could lead physicians to limit services inappropriately, resulting in inadequate care for Medicare patients. Incentive plans that shift much of the risk for services to physicians or closely tie individual treatment decisions to financial rewards pose the greatest potential threat to quality of care" (Zimmerman, Dowdal, Hultgren, and Stepek, 1988, p. 3). The incentives in the reimbursement process induce physicians to make a quality/cost trade-off, and due to their responsibility for patient care they also assume any legal consequences for the choices. Physicians are therefore placed in a difficult situation. But by pointing out the quality implications of the reimbursement processes, medicine may gain public support for more favorable payment procedures.

In light of discussions about restructuring the U.S. health care system, it is important to make a final point about physician resistance to managed care. Resistance to managed care has been relatively slight within the medical profession, and many physicians have working relationships with some form of managed care plan. However, if a radical managed care reform proposal mobilized opposition from the medical community, then physicians likely would use their relationships with patients as a basis for developing public antagonism toward the proposal. This possibility indicates the strength of the patient-provider relationship as a basis for legitimacy.

In hospitals and other traditional delivery settings, professions have had varying success at challenging the legitimacy of organizational control of employed or contracted clinical professionals. The self-governance of the medical staff in hospitals is enshrined in health care organization accrediting standards, as are requirements that credentialed professionals direct many activities. Nurses are attempting to implement a self-governance structure in many hospitals, partly as a means of asserting their independence from organizational control.

The abstract nature of professional knowledge strengthens the profession's ability to avoid "external" quality assessments, and the indetermination strategy noted in Chapter Four applies here as well. This strategy is important for employed professionals, too, as it allows them to be treated differently than other workers. As several observers have noted (for example, Sibeon, 1990), the indetermination of a profession's knowledge base can become too extreme, prompting external intervention on the grounds that the knowledge has no verifiable utility. Social work, in the eyes of some observers, has suffered from this problem. If indetermination is too low, on the other hand, the profession's work domain is subject to routinization and organizational control.

Health professions will continue to request self-governance within organizations and protection of their markets from unfettered buyer power, but their credibility will increasingly depend on their commitment to meeting stakeholders' demands for accessible, efficacious, and cost-effective care. To the extent that appeals to legislative and regulatory stakeholders are considered to be based on self-interest, they will not carry the weight they once did.

Dissemination of Price and Quality Information

Health professionals who deliver services in a fee-for-service market have had a significant advantage over buyers owing to their ability to minimize the dissemination of information about price and quality. As we shall see in Chapter Seven, internal competition restraints have included norms against advertising. Only recently has price and quality information been communicated in health professional advertising, and there still are strong norms against making public claims about quality relative to peers. Control of information about price and quality strengthens the market power of health professions over buyers, since buyers are unable to shop for better deals. Importantly, however, efforts to control such information erode the legitimacy of the professions by insinuating self-interested behavior. Demands by stakeholders for quality and price information helped stimulate the National Practitioner Data Bank and a host of consumer-oriented publications containing price and quality indicators. As buyer groups become larger and more serious about cost control, their efforts to make price and quality comparisons will accelerate. Large, organized buyers will have the staff resources to collect and monitor such information. It is in the long-term interests of health professions to accommodate rather than obfuscate these demands. Professional associations should cooperate with stakeholder organizations to provide information and encourage changing practices among their membership regarding advertising and public disclosure of prices.

Countervailing Power Through Unionization

As health care plans and third-party payers assume more power in negotiations with professionals, the building of countervailing power will become a critical strategy for health professions. This strategy entails organizing the dispersed members of a professional community into a structure that can represent the interests of the profession against a buyer possessing significant control over compensation and working conditions. In some cases, this could entail alliances among different professions facing similar relationships with buyers. The profession's organization can then wield more weight in bargaining and negotiation.

Countervailing power is an appropriate strategy when many members of a health profession derive their income from employment by a few dominant buyers. Through the exercise of monopoly or oligopoly power, the buyer frequently can control the price paid for their services. Establishing a union provides an organizational basis for the many fragmented members of the profession to build a countervailing power against the dominant employer. The union is not a seller of labor but a political institution representing the interests of the employees through collective bargaining with the dominant employer. Thus there are two distinctive bargaining entities.

Although many health professions are in the kind of market structure described above, the recent history of one profession, nursing, provides a good example of the countervailing power strategy. In the past, a small number of hospitals have dominated most market areas, and they also have cooperated in setting nursing wages. With the repeal of legal obstacles to union representation for registered nurses, unionization is a potential response to such conditions. With about one-third of hospitals having a union of some type in 1985 (Becker and Rakich, 1988), the potential for the use of union strategies is manifest. Union representation can weaken the monopoly power of hospitals, and some studies (Sloan and Steinwald, 1980; Feldman and Scheffler, 1982) confirm that such countervailing power has increased the hospital wages of nurses.

While unionization usually is perceived as a strategy used by employed health professionals, a comment about the relevance of unions to physicians is appropriate. With the growing numbers of physicians in some type of employee status, as well as the demonstrated ability of unions to increase the earnings of physicians (Liebowitz and Meyer, 1987), unions would appear to have relevance to these practitioners as a basis for undertaking a countervailing power strategy. Moreover, this potential extends beyond salaried physicians to physicians who have a contractual relationship with a managed care plan. Liebowitz and Meyer (1987, p. 44) note that for physicians in such managed care situations, "there is nothing to prevent a doctors' union from negotiating with any third party on behalf of one or more of its members, provided that antitrust laws are not breached." In addition to unionization, the following analysis suggests that joining a large-scale medical practice is another potent basis for organizing physicians against buyers such as health plans.

Compared with other health professions, the importance of physicians in producing services enhances their leverage with buyers. In an analysis of HMOs, Luft (1987, p. 318) says that "physicians control the medical process, and while other personnel and educational programs can reduce the number required, they will continue to be central figures." Events involving the Harvard Community Health Plan, a staff-model HMO, recently showed the potential power of physicians in managed care plans. Staff physicians rebelled over a proposal to link physicians' salaries to the volume of patients, causing the chief executive officer to resign. Commenting on the situation, one analyst stated that "the doctors had no idea they could bring him down" (Pastemack, 1991, p. 3). The revolt attests to the potential leverage of collective action by members of a profession whose work is especially important to the buyer.

While a strategy of countervailing power through unionization is a powerful strategic response to a dominant-employer market structure, use of the strategy raises several important issues for health professions. First, as noted in Chapter Three, many health professions attempt to acquire legitimacy through the development of scientific knowledge as a basis for their professionalization. Although unionization is one way to change the power relations between a health profession and other institutions in society, it may be viewed as undercutting the scientific status of a profession due to its "craft" connotation. Beletz (1985, p. 147), for instance, contends that representation of nurses by trade unions "destroys nurses' unique professional identity and renders them pawns designated to provide the adrenalin for the economically hurting trade unionism movement."

A second issue is exemplified by the American Nurses' Association's adherence to a "no strike" policy for eighteen years: health professions often are reluctant to use a strike to enhance their bargaining position. Strikes raise legitimacy problems with the public and, moreover, conflict with the service norm emphasizing the professional's obligation to patients. To exercise this countervailing power strategy, health professions must recognize that although nonstrike alternatives do exist (for instance, work slowdowns), a strike, or threat to strike, is probably a union's most powerful weapon.

Countervailing Power Through Professional Associations

While the exercise of countervailing power through a union is appropriate for health professions that have many members employed by a few dominant buyers, a different structural basis is more appropriate for dealing with third-party buyers who reimburse for direct service transactions between providers and patients. Professional associations can provide the structural basis for organizing members who would otherwise be fragmented in confronting the same third-party buyer.

A major example of this situation is the AMA's lobbying the federal government on behalf of physicians concerning reimbursement under Medicare. At the Medicare program's inception, the AMA's bargaining activities were instrumental in gaining the generous UCR payment system. Indeed, the system was implemented largely through private insurance carriers that were very accommodating to physicians' interests. A more recent expression of countervailing power involved proposals by the Bush administration to revise the Medicare fee schedule for physicians. When the administration sought to cut payments by several billion dollars in order to offset projected increases in the volume of services provided by physicians, lobbying by the AMA and specialty medical groups vigorously resisted payment reductions (Rich, 1991).

The pressure to contain the costs of public programs is likely to provide the federal government with a continuing incentive to exercise its monopsonistic powers to reduce reimbursement rates for clinical providers. The government has already exercised such power with regard to hospitals, reducing the annual rates of increase in DRG reimbursements in response to alleged excess profits. Glaser (1990, p. 804) has argued that the RBRVS reform in physician payments under Medicare was directed at basing reimbursement on "prices that would have resulted if the American medical services market had been truly competitive." It is unlikely, however, that conflicts among specialties and between payers and physicians can be settled by a formula determined through research, such as the RBRVS scale. Instead, Glaser believes that a negotiating system between representatives of specialty associations and the government will have an important role in determining the details of physicians' reimbursement. If such a bargaining system does emerge — with the threat of physicians' nonparticipation in Medicare serving as the analogue to a union strike — then countervailing power will be the prominent strategic response to this buyer. The strategy may require that professions propose and achieve changes in antitrust laws so they may legally share price information in order to determine bargaining positions.

Countervailing Power Through Group Practice

In addition to the traditional third-party buyers, physicians and certain independently practicing professionals face a new form of buyer: health plans. While health plans can take many forms, here we focus on those in which physicians are not employees but have a contractual relationship with the plan. These health plans have such characteristics as a directed flow of patients, risk sharing, negotiated reimbursement rates, and utilization review. The PPO and group-model HMO are examples of this kind of health plan. While the large number of such plans has mitigated their buyer power, a market shakeout could result in fewer plans with a greater potential to exercise monopoly power. Moreover, the trend for hospitals to cluster into strategic groupings in many urban health care markets (Luke, 1992) creates larger and more powerful entities whose interests are often at odds with professionals'. Consequently, health professions must devise institutional means to undertake a countervailing power strategy.

Faced with a concentrated buyer in the form of a health plan, professionals must organize into a large structural unit in order to develop the capacity to exert countervailing power. Although unionization was mentioned earlier as a possibility, at this time many health professionals prefer a more familiar structure such as a large group practice. While this analysis focuses on a group practice, other possible structural alternatives are available. The intention is to emphasize that organizing into large-scale structures yields practitioners considerable advantages in exercising countervailing power against health plans.

As a structure, large group practices offer several advantages relative to health plans. First, large groups can hire sophisticated staff to evaluate health plans and negotiate bids with the plans. Many health professionals are relatively uninformed about the criteria for evaluating the quality of the various plans. Second, large group practices can spread the risk over a larger patient base, thus reducing the risk in accepting patients from health plans. Moreover, large groups have a greater ability to diversify the source of their patients, thereby undercutting the potential leverage a health plan would derive from being the sole source of patients. Third, large groups are better able to exploit economies of scale and to hire the optimal number of auxiliary personnel in order to minimize costs. Cost minimization will be particularly important given the fixed prices of health plan contracts. And fourth, large groups have a greater capacity to develop quality assurance programs—an attractive consideration in health plan contracting.

Additional advantages of large group practices depend on the character of the practice. While antitrust ramifications must be considered, a large specialty group may be able to dominate its specialization, giving it market power relative to a health plan. In this situation, particular attention must be given to relationships with primary care practitioners because they will be an important source of patient referrals that diversify the group's patient base. In contrast to the specialty group practice, a multispecialty practice provides an internal solution to the referral problem. This is attractive not only for purposes of diversifying the patient base but also because it gives the practice a degree of control over a major difficulty in managed care: specialist referral.

While this analysis focuses on a large group practice as a structure, there is also a potential *interorganizational* advantage to this form of practice. Large groups, which are a valued source of patients to hospitals, can gain many advantages from a formal relationship with a hospital. Groups can use the expertise that hospitals have accumulated in negotiating managed care contracts, essentially "transferring overhead" from the group to the hospital (Coddington, Keen, Moore, and Clarke, 1990, p. 54). And through formal relationships with hospitals, such as joint ventures or regional specialty centers, the large group gains a major institutional ally in bargaining with the health plans.

Finally, large group practices will have to monitor product differentiation among health plans. Future health plans are likely to develop beyond their current homogeneous character of generalized price discounting: differentiation may well emerge along quality/cost dimensions (Coddington, Keen, Moore, and Clarke, 1990). In such a segmented market, group practices can gain leverage by promoting themselves as able to meet the particular needs of a particular health plan.

Ownership of Health Plans

While a strategy of countervailing power is one strategic response to health plans as a buyer, professionals can also adopt a competition strategy. In this scenario, the professionals themselves form a health plan — thereby assuming responsibility for providing both the insurance and the service. They then market their plan directly to buyers such as employers, government, and individual consumers. The delivery structure can assume a variety of forms such as independent practice associations (IPAs), large group practices, or joint ventures between various groups such as physicians, psychologists, optometrists, nurses, physical therapists, hospitals, laboratories, and pharmacies. Essentially the competition strategy eliminates the health plan's role as a coordinator. The strategy thus becomes a way to retain professional autonomy rather than submitting to contractual constraints imposed by a nonprofessionally owned health plan. In provider-owned plans, providers are able to use "the unique knowlege and inside relationships with peers that outside parties do not have" to create flexible and responsive systems (Heintz and McNerney, 1992, p. 23).

Provider-owned health plans can assuage professionals' concerns about autonomy and still result in domination of a market area, particularly rural locales (Coddington, Keen, Moore, and Clarke, 1990). Their success, however, will depend on the competitiveness of the marketplace and the attractiveness of the product to the direct buyers of health plans. Physicians formed IPAs as a competitive response to staff-model and group-model HMOs, and they have learned that strategic success depends on their pricing structure relative to utilization and reimbursement rates. The managed care system that can balance these variables best is most likely to have the greatest market success — regardless of its sponsorship.

Bridging Strategies

Another basic strategy for influencing buyers is for members of a health profession to become participants in the buyer organization. By assuming positions in management and on governing boards, consultative committees, and salary committees, they can influence decisions about reimbursement and working conditions of professionals. While this bridging strategy may entail bargaining at some point, it differs from the countervailing power strategy in that the latter involves negotiations between two distinct organizational entities: the buyer and the one representing the profession's members. The bridging strategy highlights the potential for influence based on gaining certain roles in the buyer's organizational structure.

A good example of this strategy is the historic relationship between Blue Shield and physicians. Physicians always have been concerned that insurance companies, as third parties to the financial transaction between doctors and patients, could have interests that conflict with the medical community's. Insurers might substitute conservative reimbursement methods, update reimbursement rates infrequently, restrict the scope of covered services, or implement rigorous review of utilization. Generally, an insurer with a large volume could exercise monopsonistic market power to negotiate price discounts, thereby lowering physicians' incomes.

To avoid the potentially adverse effects of third-party involvement in insurance while still retaining the income advantages of insuring services, physicians sought to control Blue Shield through participation on the boards of directors. With various qualifications, different empirical analyses (Arnould and Eisenstadt, 1981; Kass and Pautler, 1981) have concluded that physicians' influence on the boards of directors resulted in higher reimbursement for physicians. Feldstein (1988a) and Starr (1982) argue that various characteristics of the method of reimbursement facilitated monopoly power over the pricing of physician services. In essence, participation on the boards led to such strong influence that bargaining with Blue Shield was unnecessary.

The case of Blue Shield underscores the potential value of involvement in a payer organization. It should be noted, however, that it is an extreme example because state and county medical societies formed Blue Shield plans. Following a critical Federal Trade Commission analysis, the Blue Shield plans eliminated physician-controlled boards (Greenberg, 1991), making it necessary for physicians to seek other sources of structural influence. Physicians' involvement on committees for peer review, fee schedules, and utilization review may provide such access points for influence in the future.

While this example focuses on physicians and Blue Shield, it is important to note that two rapidly growing payers—HMOs and PPOs—also provide opportunities for the exercise of an organizational bridging strategy. Physician consensus committees within HMOs and PPOs review relative value scales for possible modification in light of resource costs for the production of services (Ogrod and Doherty, 1988, p. 90). Some analysts believe that the promise of cost containment by organized health plans is foundering. Physicians' participation "in the design of the product, the marketing plan, and the quality assurance and cost monitoring process," they say, could solidify the plans' viability (Coddington, Keen, Moore, and Clarke, 1990, p. 200). Physicians in one of Minneapolis–St. Paul's largest HMOs, Physicians Health Plan, successfully fought for representation on the organization's board—and reimbursement rates were a major issue that prompted the fight (Rundle, 1987). While such roles are not as powerful as dominating a board of directors, they do provide an opportunity for health professions to influence a payer's decision-making processes concerning reimbursement.

Sometimes the small number of professional employees undercuts the possibility of a countervailing power strategy. Employees of solo physicians, group medical practices, and home health agencies find that the structural balance of power favors the employer. In the absence of an external structure (for example, a union) to represent their interests, members of a health profession in this situation will have to use an organizational strategy that exerts pressure on the internal management practices. In this case, emphasis on the professionals' contribution to the firm's productivity is probably the strongest negotiating position to assume in relation to the buyer. Studies have established the contribution of auxiliary personnel to the productivity of physician and dental practices (Smith, Miller, and Golladay, 1972; Reinhardt, 1974). While the amount of income generated by nurse practitioners and physician assistants for medical practices depends on the type of physician, evidence shows that the profitability ratio of these practitioners is relatively high (Johnson and Cawley, 1991). Indeed, the income generated by such practitioners increased at a faster rate than the costs—indicating a very favorable contribution to the employer's productivity. Members of many health professions could use this state of affairs to legitimate their claims with such employers.

The growing proportion of professionals who are employed by large organizations reinforces the need to attain greater influence on management practices. There are several strategies to achieve influence: creating administrative subcommunities within each of the clinical health professions (as medicine, pharmacy, and nursing have done) and pressuring organizations and accreditors of organizations to allow or even require professional representation in the management of groups of professionals. Professional communities can encourage or provide management education for clinical professionals to give them the expertise to serve as managers. Even more crucial is participation at the top level of the organization — on executive management teams or on boards.

Participation in management gives the profession a voice in critical issues that affect its competitive position relative to the organization. This is particularly important given the conflict between the traditional autonomy needs of professionals and the new "total quality management" philosophies that emphasize collective responsibility and accountability of all organizational participants (McLaughlin and Kaluzny, 1990). The ability of health professionals to influence management practices will depend on their negotiating power within the organization (Bacharach, Bamberger, and Conley, 1991).

A similar bridging with buyers' concerns is exhibited when health professions expand their education to include knowledge on cost-effectiveness and other buyer concerns, such as ethical issues. The profession's demonstration of concern lends credibility to the argument that it cares about the problems of buyers.

Alternative Buyers

Since the organizational bridging strategy can be used by members of health professions who derive income either from employers or service transactions, bridging strategies have broad applicability. Regardless of the type of transaction, efforts can be made to influence reimbursement and other management decisions by gaining positions within the buyer's organization. Another strategy, however, applies to a narrower class of practitioners — those who derive their income from service transactions. The focus of this strategy is for independent practitioners to receive their income from *many* diverse buyers.

One reason for the diversification strategy concerns the provider's vulnerability to the buyer's power. If a provider receives a large proportion of income from a particular buyer, then he or she is vulnerable to the power of the buyer in the same way that employed professionals are. To avoid the "sole source" situation faced by salaried employees, independent practitioners can try to develop a buyer base that provides a multiple-source income stream. Such a situation minimizes the leverage that any single buyer can exert over the practitioner. According to this logic, providers should support fragmentation in the health plan market and avoid committing themselves to any one plan.

Apart from reducing a provider's vulnerability to the buyer's power, diversification opens the possibility of shifting costs. Independent practitioners receiving income from service transactions are likely to experience some degree of nonpayment and relatively low payment rates from fixed-fee buyers such as Medicare, Medicaid, and managed care plans. It may be possible to compensate for nonpayment and low rates by shifting costs to fee-for-service, self-pay, and IPA patients. While cost shifting has a compensatory effect, this strategy may be self-defeating in the long run if victimized buyers push for preventive regulations or a uniform payment system develops.

The mention of self-pay patients suggests another point. In contrast with major buyers, the balance of power in relationships with self-pay patients usually has favored the health professions, particularly physicians and dentists. Historically, domination has been rooted in the consumer's ignorance of the quality of the product (for example, dental or medical care), failure of consumers to price shop, and the ability of the professions to control internal competition. Professionals have been able to gain higher incomes from these buyers than if there were a freely competitive market.

The utility of maximizing the quantity of self-pay patients is likely to diminish in the future. First, the proportion of health care spending from self-pay patients is decreasing. Second, consumer ignorance and cartel constraints are declining in importance with the emergence and enhanced legitimacy of a competitive approach to health care (Feldstein, 1988a; Pauly, 1988). Third, there are limits to the extent of cost shifting that self-pay patients will accept — and these limits may have already been reached in many markets.

Gaming Strategies

A final note regarding relationships with buyers concerns the professional's ability to manipulate reimbursement systems. Gaming strategies are available to all health professions regardless of the method of reimbursement. Gaming involves manipulating, interpreting, and adapting to the payment process in a way that is advantageous to the income goals of the health profession. The possibility of gaming arises from the presumption, noted by natural systems theorists (Scott, 1992), that no formal system of rules can completely control behavior. While rules may be established with a particular intent, human behavior, stemming from cynical calculations or otherwise, can undermine that intent or create unintended consequences.

The fee-for-service reimbursement of physicians provides illustrative examples of gaming. Fee-for-service gives physicians an incentive to provide more services in order to increase their incomes. There are, moreover, gaming responses to fee freezes and fee reductions designed to control cost escalation: increasing the volume of services, changing the mix, labeling, and site of the services (Eisenberg, 1986), as well as fragmenting integrated services into discrete parts (Feldstein, 1988a). Indeed, other analysts have noted that vertical integration—that is, expanding the mix of services by adding "advanced office-based diagnostic equipment, outpatient surgery, or downstream services such as physical therapy"—was a major way that physicians boosted their incomes in the past decade (Coddington, Keen, Moore, and Clarke, 1990, p. 221). The RBRVS reimbursement process of Medicare may become vulnerable to such gaming strategies, as well, with induced volume, substitution of services, and "RBRVS creep" emerging as possible adaptive responses of the medical profession.

Salary and capitation reimbursement methods are also subject to gaming strategies. Once a salary has been determined, a major gaming variable under the control of employees is the quantity and quality of their work. A quantitative gaming response to salary dissatisfaction takes the form of limiting the amount of work performed; qualitative gaming is expressed through routine, mediocre work. In his analysis of physicians' satisfaction in HMOs, Luft (1987) alludes to this kind of adaptive behavior, warning that high workloads damage the quality of the physician/patient interaction. From an economic perspective, quantitative and qualitative gaming can be viewed as ways for salaried employees to reduce the work per dollar of pay.

The gaming responses to capitation payment are similar to those in salary reimbursement. While there is a great variety of capitation arrangements in managed care plans, there is generally an incentive to underserve the patient. The lower the quantity of services, the higher the reimbursement for the provider. If the plan allows the opportunity, the provider may even consider "offloading" expensive patients to other providers. There is also an incentive to reduce the quality of services to capitated patients, especially in comparison to the provider's fee-for-service patients.

A major problem with gaming strategies is that they can diminish legitimacy and invite more severe intervention if the intended effects of the original intervention are not realized. The volume performance standards in Medicare's new RBRVS reimbursement program for physicians suggest that the federal government is ready to move against such gaming activities. Gaming diminishes legitimacy because providers are seen as enhancing their own incomes, a particularly risky situation. Americans are angry about the incomes of certain providers, even though they underestimate actual incomes ("Health Industry High Pay Angers Citizens, Poll Finds," 1993). Providers are vulnerable to the "special interest" label, which helps explain why a majority of voters support a national health insurance program if it is financed by taxation of health service providers (Blendon and others, 1992). The provider's incentives to pursue a gaming strategy can be quite high, however, so it may take extensive educational efforts by professional associations to convince their members that gaming is not in the long-term strategic interest of the community.

Conventional and Contemporary Strategies

Changes in the buyer sector of health services represent the newest and most significant strategic challenge to many of the health professions. Yet changes in the buyer sector also offer opportunities for many professions. To manage these challenges and opportunities, health professions should consider the contempo-

Table 6.1. Strategies for Managing Relationships with Buyers.

Conventional Strategies

- Control the supply of services by requiring licensing, promoting specialty certification, standardizing education, inhibiting substitution, and discouraging internal competition.
- Generate demand for services by gaining direct reimbursement from third-party payers and expanding the work domain.
- Combat buyer power through legal means and claims to defend the patient/provider relationship.
- Discourage dissemination of price and quality information.
- Gain a voice in the governance of employer organizations and third-party payer organizations through technical expertise and claims to represent the patient's interest.
- Maximize the proportion of clients who self-pay.
- Pursue gaming tactics to maximize income.

Contemporary Strategies

- Assure an adequate supply of practitioners to meet society's demands.
- Generate demand for services by expanding diversity of settings and identifying and meeting the needs of new market segments.
- Accommodate buyers' demands for price and quality information.
- Build countervailing power structures to offset the negotiating power of large organized buyers.
- Form provider-owned and managed health plans to compete with other health plans.
- Gain a voice in the governance of employer organizations through contributions to organizational productivity.

rary strategies listed in Table 6.1. These strategies center on better response to the demands of buyers for accessible, cost-effective, and efficacious services, along with innovative organization in the marketplace to counteract the power of large buyer organizations. Efforts to expand the demand for services should take advantage of demographic trends, illness patterns, and the decentralization of delivery settings.

These new strategies contrast with the conventional strategies for managing relationships with buyers compiled in Table 6.1. Conventional strategies, which emphasize defensive measures designed to avoid rather than accommodate buyer demands, will no longer enable the health professions to meet their long-term goals. Health professions must come to terms with the growing power of buyers — employers, insurers, and consumers — to shape the workplace environment and the reward structure of professional work.

Chapter Seven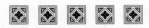

Internal Organization and Management

Much of the strategic activity of the professional community is concerned with relationships with external stakeholders: substitutes, buyers, suppliers, and regulators. But strategic adaptation also requires that professional communities manage relationships with their internal stakeholders — the individual professionals and associations that comprise the community.

At the most basic level, professional communities must have a certain degree of integration or the community no longer exists except as a collection of separate individuals. As discussed in Chapter Two, professional communities are differentiated into segments based on geography, specialty, level of education, and many other characteristics. The individuals and associations within the community must communicate and unite if coordinated action in the pursuit of community goals is to take place. Business firms do not face a challenge of this magnitude, as the employment relationship creates formal bonds among people and daily interaction among employees is extensive. Professional communities, however, must devote significant resources to overcoming differentiation.

Another basic internal challenge for the professional community is to create structures and management practices that are consistent with strategies. A new countervailing power strategy toward organized buyers, for example, might require that the community adopt a more cooperative attitude and more coordinated organizational structures. A strategy of diversifying the profession's work domain might entail new organizational arrangements that encourage the development of members' knowledge and entrepreneurial spirit. New structures and management practices may cause dissent within the community, however, such that bold action to overcome conflict may become necessary in concert with the implementation of changes.

In order to alter their internal structure, professions can manipulate their size, composition, knowledge base, culture, and organization — the key internal dimensions of professional communities introduced in Chapter Two (along with differentiation and collective goals). In this chapter we discuss the issues of management and organization as they relate to these major internal dimensions. The chapter ends with a discussion of the management of change in professional communities.

Managing Size and Composition

As explained in Chapter Six, size is an important strategic tool of the professional community, for the size of the profession relative to demand influences its continuing legitimacy and market power. The management of size in relation to demand is a complex undertaking. Overall size may have little meaning in highly specialized professions. Indeed, many observers contend that the United States is oversupplied with many types of physician specialists but undersupplied with primary care physicians. Another complication in managing size is the existence of profession-induced demand — that is, the ability of professionals to create demand by their mere presence. The implication of profession-induced demand is that buyers may in fact require fewer professionals than they appear to demand in the market. A third complication relates to the geographic dispersion of professionals: one geographic area may be oversupplied, another undersupplied.

These complications do not obviate the need for extensive monitoring, forecasting, and efforts to manage supply by professional communities. Market forces and other factors so far seem unable to adequately govern the supply of physicians, nurses, or allied health personnel. Indeed, major shortages or oversupplies are declared sporadically but chronically in virtually all the health professions. This situation inevitably leads to greater external intervention in the educational process in order to manage the geographic location, specialization, and total supply of practitioners. As Ginzberg (1992, p. 3118) warns regarding physician supply: "If the medical establishment fails to act, others will act, and the results are likely to be less satisfactory for all concerned." An important dimension of a strategy of responding to buyer demands is the management of supply.

Managing size is complicated by the imperfect integration of the educational subcommunity and other stakeholders into the profession. Educational institutions and training sites often have incentives to maintain or increase the size of classes. Specialty certification and educational accreditation organizations have incentives to do the same. Communication and coordination among the associations and groups that influence supply are necessary for effective management of size.

The professional community's internal dimensions include the distribution of members by personal attributes such as race, ethnicity, and gender. Of particular concern here is the racial and gender composition of the profession. Historically, the most successful health professions have been overwhelmingly composed of white males. Demands that the most rewarding health careers be accessible to all racial and ethnic groups and to both genders emanate from the social value of equity and from a desire for health care that responds to the needs of subgroups in our society. The implication that health professions which are disproportionately white and male should begin to promote racial and gender diversity is controversial, but it is an important issue that professional communities must face. Again, external intervention is likely if they do not.

A final management issue deserves mention here. To the extent that members' personal attributes determine the professional community's goals and its access to resources, the community must recognize those attributes. An example is the possibility that "deferential, obsequious attitudes" engendered by female socialization reduce the desire of female-dominated health professions to pursue confrontational strategies (Styles, 1982, p. 19). There are two possible responses to such patterns affecting strategic adaptation: attempt to change the attitudes and behavior, or pursue strategies that acknowledge the attitudes and behavior. Contemporary nursing seems to be pursuing the first approach (Roberts, 1983).

Managing the Knowledge Base

Previous chapters have depicted the critical role that management of a profession's knowledge base plays in the attainment of legitimacy and market power. By definition of the profession itself, the knowledge base plays an even more critical role — it links together the individual members of the profession. The knowledge base is the central integrating element of the professional community's structure. To the extent that individuals share a common knowledge base, they are bonded to each other. This requires that the community exert control over the knowledge base and its evolution.

Historically, management of the knowledge base has been pursued by vertical integration of two important sets of stakeholders into the professional community: teachers and researchers. If we view professional communities as having inputs (individual practitioners) and outputs (health services), the vertical integration of teachers and researchers internalizes the control of inputs to the community. Standardization and control of the flow of inputs to the community becomes much easier to attain. Management of the flow of teachers and educators is important in managing *access* to the knowledge base and continuing *development* of the knowledge base. A third area of strategic concern is *application* of the knowledge base in the work setting. Strategies for managing the knowledge base at all three points are presented next.

Standardization and Control of Entry Education

As conveyed in Chapter Three, a key step in the process of attaining legitimacy for health professions has been the standardization and control of entry to the profession. As noted, most of the health professions have essentially integrated into the professional community the producers of new entrants to the profession. If integration of the entry organizations is complete, the teachers of the new entrants are members of the profession and educational facilities are accredited by the professional community itself, giving the profession control over length of education and content of curricula. State laws typically specify the entry requirements for the profession, and they are enforced largely by a profession-dominated state licensing board. In these ways, standardization of entry education has facilitated the profession's achievement of legitimacy.

The same strategy has important ramifications for integration of the professional community. Vertical integration of the entry education process means that all members share the bonds of a common educational experience. They, and only they, become competent to judge the quality of their peers' work. To the extent that these members share a common knowledge base, a strong bond is created, even if they acquire additional knowledge for their own specialty areas. While medicine is highly specialized, for example, all members of the community share a common knowledge base imparted in medical school.

If standardization of entry education is incomplete, entrants can more easily become a source of internal stratification or disintegration. The fact that registered nurses enter the profession through several different educational paths has potent effects on community integration. Registered nurses are quite aware of distinctions among those educated in hospital diploma, associate degree, and four-year-college settings. A great deal of energy, emotion, and other resources have been expended by segments of registered nursing in their failed efforts to standardize entry education at the baccalaureate level (Kovner, 1990). Pharmacists face internal schisms among those whose entry credential is the relatively new Pharm.D. degree, which requires one year more of study (a total of six years of college) than the older baccalaureate entry degree. Multiple educational pathways into health care administration, such as the M.S., M.H.A., M.P.H., and M.B.A. degrees, create internal friction within that profession (Pointer, Luke, and Brown, 1986). Even when professionals receive the same educational credential, differences in their curricula may impede integration. In the recent past, for example, three of the seventeen schools of chiropractic were accredited by the Straight Chiropractic Academic Standards Association, which held a conservative view of the chiropractor's scope of work domain, rather than the Council on Chiropractic Education, which held a more expansive view (U.S. Department of Health and Human Services, 1992).

Integration of educators and educational organizations into the professional community is not easy to attain or maintain. In the first place, educational organizations may arise outside the practitioner community. For-profit or proprietary schools have existed in many of the health professions, and their allegiance to investors may conflict with the interests of the professional community. The Flexner Report in medicine, noted in Chapter Six, was highly critical of proprietary medical schools. Another potential source of educational programs is the employers of health professionals. Hospitals have been the initiators of educational programs in many of the health professions, such as medical technology and radiologic technology. Registered nurses have long been educated by hospital diploma programs. Large hospital chains such as Humana and large HMOs such as Kaiser Permanente have their own training programs for many health professionals. Again, the concerns of employers may diverge from those of practitioners, hindering the professional community's efforts to control its knowledge base.

Even if the professional community does successfully integrate entry educators, the potential for conflict between educators and practitioners remains, due to their differing goals. Teachers are more likely to emphasize new knowledge, for example, and to direct students toward specialization and toward academic rather than practice concerns. As we shall see later in this chapter, practitioners may support a downsizing of the new entrant pool, while educators may not. Thus tension is inherent in the relationship between educators and practitioners. The history of medical education is fraught with such strains, as practitioners have battled medical educators over access to private patients, educators' lack of orientation to the community, and educators' research orientations (Kendall, 1965; Ludmerer, 1985). Separating clinical and basic science departments in medical schools is one way medicine has attempted to accommodate disparate educational, research, and practice interests.

Changes in the level of entry education required can hamper integration — particularly if educational curricula change significantly and members educated under the former entry curriculum do not identify with those educated under the new one. Pharmacy's attempt to upgrade entry-level education is a source of divisiveness within the professional community. The raising of standards — often the result of a push for greater legitimacy and market power — may be undertaken at the sacrifice (at least in the short term) of integration.

Continuing Development of the Knowledge Base

Vertical integration of educational institutions into the professional community facilitates the continuing development of new knowledge within the profession's "paradigm" or philosophy of practice. Integration is expedited if members themselves develop the new knowledge that is passed on to new and existing members. Thus researchers and research organizations that are loyal to the professional community should be developed inside the community or should be courted if they are outside the community.

Health professions commonly strive to develop within the professional community a cadre of doctorally prepared researchers who share the basic values of the practitioner. Typically, the doctoral degrees may be attained in fields outside the profession until the profession develops its own doctoral programs — as, for instance, physical therapy and nursing recently have done. Many of these doctorally prepared researchers are expected to do research for the benefit of the practicing members of the professional community. In addition, control over research reinforces control of the teaching function, as teaching and research frequently are performed by the same people and organizations. To the extent that the development of new knowledge is under the profession's control, it can influence the type of research conducted and, in some ways, the dissemination of research findings. Changes in the profession's knowledge base, then, can be developed with consideration for the effects on the practitioner community as a whole.

Most health professions also sponsor research journals, aiding control over the dissemination of research and the type of research performed, to the extent that researchers depend on publication in these journals for their own career advancement. As is the case with control of entry education, there is a danger that control over the development of new knowledge can isolate the profession from developments outside its boundaries or its paradigm. The profession becomes more vulnerable to external forces if it is totally buffered from sources of new knowledge outside the community. Dissent and criticism of the professional paradigm may be stifled by nonpublication of important ideas, leading the community to ignore crucial external pressures.

Competitors for control over the research function include proprietary enterprises such as firms that supply products used in the delivery of health services. One study has estimated that private industry's funding of biomedical research has grown from 32 percent in 1950 to 42 percent in 1987 (Ginzberg and Dutka, 1989). A large complex of commercial biotechnology firms in the United States and elsewhere conducts research on genes that could have dramatic implications for treatment of the health problems addressed by most of the health professions. Suppliers of medical technology conduct research to develop new machines and products that change practice patterns of health professionals. The development of outpatient surgical techniques, for example, has affected the work domain of hospital administrators by creating new competitors for their organizations. Pharmacy represents a professional community that incompletely encompasses the development of new knowledge. Large pharmaceutical companies explicitly influence the direction and speed of research by funding research and employing researchers, many of whom do not hold pharmacy degrees. Finally, health care delivery organizations seek to gain market power by developing new treatment techniques. Several large hospital firms now advertise treatments developed by "their" health professionals.

Another growing source of new knowledge is the purchasers of health services, including employers and insurance
companies and governments. The constantly increasing cost of
medical care has led to the formation of a vast complex of health
services researchers studying the cost-effectiveness of clinical
treatments, sometimes with only marginal involvement by the
affected professions. The FTC, for instance, on behalf of the
buyers of visionwear, studied the cost and quality of eyeglasses
and contact lenses in the 1970s and 1980s despite noncoopera-
tion from many of the involved professions. The Agency for
Health Care Policy and Research was directed by 1989 legislation to develop and assess clinical practice guidelines for health
professionals, and its Medical Treatment Effectiveness Program
has sponsored a wide range of studies of clinical treatment effectiveness, as well as dissemination of treatment guidelines (U.S.
Department of Health and Human Services, 1991). The Food
and Drug Administration and the Congressional Office of Technology Assessment are active in the assessment of health product
and service effectiveness, too. In the provider sector, insurance
companies such as Blue Cross and Blue Shield, and large-scale
providers such as Intermountain Health Care and U.S. Healthcare, sponsor treatment effectiveness research—as do private
foundations such as the Robert Wood Johnson Foundation and
the Commonwealth Fund, as well as provider associations such
as the Academic Medical Centers Consortium. The role of such
organizations outside the affected professions is likely to continue to grow in the future (Field and Lohr, 1992; Perry and
Pillar, 1990).

In general, while control over entry education and the
development of new knowledge by the professional community
facilitates integration, such control can lead to neglect of buyers'
needs as well as changes in knowledge and technology that are
outside the profession's educational paradigm or at the margin.
Internalization of the research function is counterproductive
when it encourages the profession to ignore the interests of
powerful buyers, as it can prompt outside intervention. For instance, Light (1988, p. 308) has argued that "medical schools
and their training institutions find themselves no longer the in-
spiration and source of advance for a professionally driven system

but an impediment and a source of frustration for a buyer-driven system." The failure of educators to teach clinical health profession students about the cost and access implications of their practice patterns prompted the assessment that health professional training and education are "out of step with the evolving health needs of the American people" and that education should teach practitioners to "incorporate and balance cost and quality in the decision-making process" (Shugars, O'Neil, and Bader, 1991, pp. iii, 19). Regulators and buyers are questioning the professional community's control of the education program accreditation process, as well.

If the management of knowledge is to be more responsive to the demands of buyers, professional communities must vigorously intervene in the work domains of their members through the development and dissemination of practice guidelines. This is by no means easy or noncontroversial, as it sets up new conflicts between specialties or between believers in one style of practice versus another. Freidson (1985) expects that internal conflict among practitioners, physician-administrators, and physician-researchers over norms of clinical practice will be a major problem for the medical profession. In dentistry, the ability of the American Dental Association to issue practice guidelines was challenged by certain practitioners and a sub-community association (the American Academy of Head, Facial and Neck Pain and TMJ Disorders) as a restraint on trade in the case of electronic devices used to diagnose temporomandibular joint disorders (Goodman, 1990).

Yet if professional communities do not develop practice guidelines, government and buyer groups will. Professions can join and influence research efforts that affect their practice domain. Alternatively, they can attempt to perform the assessment functions themselves or take the lead in doing so. The American Medical Association, for example, has worked with the Rand Corporation to develop clinical guidelines in several areas of care, while the American College of Physicians has promulgated treatment guidelines itself. Many health professions are encouraging research training for members of their profession in order to enhance the profession's ability to conduct the research itself.

Dissemination of new knowledge to experienced practitioners is an important management task of the professional community. Historically, the need to maintain integration in the face of changes in the knowledge base has resulted in the common practice of "grandfathering"—exempting current practitioners from new educational requirements for licensure or other credentials. Grandfathering coopts those in the profession who do not share the new knowledge. Grandfathering can raise legitimacy concerns, however, as buyers and regulators may question why new members of the professional community need certain knowledge but veteran members do not. These concerns assume more weight today than they did in the past.

The professions increasingly will need to bridge with relevant suppliers of knowledge and technology in order to identify early signs of obsolescence of professional tasks and continually upgrade the education and skills of practitioners after their initial education. Formal continuing education is a means of smoothing the flow of new information into the profession so it can be digested by practitioners. Many health professions require members to receive continuing education that meets specified standards in order for them to qualify for relicensure. Annual conferences and research journals stockpile and package new information so that it can be more economically transmitted to practitioners. Professions will need to emphasize lifelong learning, rather than initial entry education, and pay greater attention to recertifying and reexamining practitioners over the years. Through these mechanisms, members of the community can keep up with the changing knowledge base and will be less likely to oppose changes in the profession's direction.

Application of the Knowledge Base

Professions also have a strategic interest in controlling the *application* of their knowledge base in the work setting. This effort often involves dealing with employers, a topic covered in more detail in Chapter Six due to its relevance to market power. In this section we relate the issue of work settings to integration of the community.

At one extreme, members of a professional community may primarily be self-employed — as is the case in dentistry, medicine, optometry, and certain other health professions. Self-employment minimizes the strains that are created by pressure from employers to act in ways inimical to the profession's interests. At the other extreme are the professions in which almost all members are employed, such as medical technology and radiologic technology. To the extent that employment settings create different interests, integration of the professional community is threatened. Hospital pharmacists, for example, have different goals than community pharmacists. Optometrists employed in retail outlets have had quite different goals than self-employed optometrists. Administrators employed in long-term-care facilities have interests so different from administrators employed in acute facilities that the two usually are identified as distinct professions. The splintering of interests based on diversity of employment setting is a major challenge for the health professions.

Another challenge arises when a work activity can be routinized such that it can be performed by lower-level employees. This, of course, can occur in both employed and self-employed work settings. In both cases, the profession may seek to create a lower level of personnel over which it retains control. The superior/subordinate relationship may be codified in licensing laws and control of educational program accreditation, as is the case with medicine's superordinate relationship with many of the allied health professions.

Subordinate professions may or may not remain organizationally within the professional community of the superior. Medical record technicians, for instance, belong to the same primary professional association as their superiors in the workplace, medical record administrators. The same is true for occupational therapy assistants and occupational therapists, as well as for physical therapy assistants and physical therapists. In some cases, though, the interests of the subordinate group are quite different than those of the superior and the goal of integration may not be well served by the forced alliance of the two groups. Examples are physician assisting, which is organized independently of medicine, and dental hygiene, which is organized separately from dentistry. The professional community of pharmacy currently is debating the wisdom of developing pharmacy technicians inside or outside the professional community of pharmacists.

It is difficult to generalize about trends in the development of subordinate professions. On the one hand, if subordinate professions can substitute for independent professions, they may be more cost-effective than the alternative — a combination of two "independent" or less hierarchically ordered professions. This is the argument that physicians used in the 1980s for creation of a new professional, the registered care technician (RCT), who would work under the authority of the physician. The physician-RCT combination would be more cost-effective than the physician–nurse combination, medicine argued, and on those grounds the proposal was attractive to employers of health professionals.

On the other hand, subordination reduces the possibility that the subordinate can substitute for the superior profession, in contrast to independent practice of the "subordinate." This, for example, gives employers an incentive to oppose subordination of the pharmacy technician to the pharmacist. In general, it is likely that hierarchical control will not be supported by external stakeholders of a profession unless it is cost-effective, as noted in Chapter Four on substitute relationships. In any event, the health professions can expect a growing number of suggestions for rearranging work boundaries (or making boundaries more flexible) in order to accommodate innovation in the division of labor — whether the proposals involve new subordinate professions or the creation of substitutes.

When subordinate professions are retained within the professional community, it is important that their work satisfaction be sustained, lest they become a force for disintegration within the professional community. One way of doing this is to create career ladders offering opportunities for movement upward to the superordinate profession. This measure has the added benefit of creating a ready source of new recruits to the profession.

In summary, then, employment relationships can challenge the integration of a professional community. And these challenges are likely to be of increasing concern in the future as organizations attempt to extend their managerial control over professionals. Yet the ability of professions to meet the demands of their employer stakeholders will be an increasing component of their successful strategic adaptation, as was argued in Chapter Six. To cope with these challenges, professions also will need to educate their members and prepare them for change, a topic we cover at the end of this chapter.

Managing Internal Culture

Knowledge is imparted to the professional within the context of the profession's culture—the shared norms, values, beliefs, and assumptions of the members. In recent years, business organizations have come to recognize the importance of their internal culture in developing strategic strength (Ulrich and Lake, 1991). The instillment of a common professional culture in members of a profession is important for its integrative effects, and the content of that culture shapes the strategies pursued by the profession.

A broad and deep professional culture has the ability to cross both horizontal and vertical lines of differentiation within the profession. Breadth of culture is the degree to which all members share a basic set of norms and values. Depth refers to the degree to which professional norms and values are adhered to in daily work life. Commitment to norms and values can be superficial or deep. In strong professional cultures members not only share the same type of work. They draw their identity from that work, share beliefs that extend beyond work matters, and meld work and leisure in their social relationships (Van Maanen and Barley, 1984).

Initial and Continuing Socialization

Organizations with strong cultures expose their new employees to extensive socialization. Thus a common strategy for strengthening the breadth and depth of internal culture is to increase the length of the initial educational period. In professions that tightly manage the initial educational experience, through accreditation and control over the credentialing of teachers, the creation of a strong culture is easier. Most nursing schools encourage or even require their new faculty members to have doctoral degrees in nursing rather than related fields in an effort to manage the culture of the educational institutions as well as the development of new knowledge.

To the extent that the initial socialization experience is special or unique, its bonding effects are enhanced. Rites and ceremonies — such as the "pinning" of nurses and the administration of the Hippocratic Oath to physicians upon graduation — underscore the special nature of the achievement of the initial credential. Medical school and residency training are renowned for their rigor and their demeaning treatment of students. The powerful effects of medical school socialization have been chronicled in detail (Becker, Geer, Hughes, and Strauss, 1961; Konner, 1987), and most of the other health professions have adopted a similar strategy of immersing students in full-time intensive study, often under stressful conditions. Completion of postentry certification requirements in many of the health professions is an onerous, time-consuming process as well. Achievement of fellowship status in the American College of Healthcare Executives can take about ten years, for example, with continuous membership, written and oral examinations, and a written project required along with continuing education, leadership, and service expectations. But completion of these onerous processes, whether initial or postentry, reinforces the notion that graduates are special and are entering a club whose nature outsiders will never fully comprehend.

Another strategy for instilling professional values is to require study of the profession's history and traditions during the initial education period. Curricula in many health professions include a course that explores the historical development of the profession. Such courses ingrain the notion that the profession has had a unique and important role over a long time period — thereby inspiring deep commitment. Professions with strong cultures nurture their history. They celebrate important occasions such as founders' days. They memorialize heroes, such as William Osler in medicine, Andrew Taylor Still in osteopathy, or Florence Nightingale in nursing, through the naming of awards or clubs or journals. Professions with a long history can draw upon traditions that have persisted over the years. An example is the Hippocratic Oath in medicine, which dates from the fifth century B.C.

Similarly, initial education may include exposure to the primary professional association and its code of ethics. Student chapters of professional associations are an important facet of this strategy, and educational programs often sponsor student chapters of professional associations. The primary association's code of ethics promulgates the basic philosophy of the profession, and it may be discussed in coursework during the initial socialization period.

Later socialization experiences, subsequent to initial education and training, can contribute to maintaining (or altering) the professional culture. Meetings of associations, continuing education offerings, journals, and newsletters all enable a professional community to share (or change) common norms and values. But only in the initial educational process are attendance and attention requisite, so these later activities often reinforce prior beliefs rather than develop new allegiance to the profession.

Codes of ethics and licensing laws contain norms that are expected to govern behavior after the initial socialization period. Important aspects of a profession's internal culture are expressed in the code of ethics of the primary professional association, to which members of the profession, particularly those who belong to the primary association, are expected to adhere. A typical code espouses norms for both personal and professional behavior. The code of ethics of the American College of Healthcare Executives, for example, commits members to "conduct all personal and professional activities with honesty, integrity, respect, fairness, and good faith." They should work with other members to "enhance the dignity and image of the healthcare management profession." Moreover, service goals usually are promulgated — as in the ACHE code's pledge for executives to "work to identify and meet the healthcare needs of the community" and "work to assure that all people have reasonable access to healthcare services" (Neuhauser, 1990). Historically, the behavior of all health care practitioners "was supposed to be oriented toward the provision of humane care in which biomedical knowledge would be applied to benefit patients and communities, even if this required departures from economically rational behavior" (Gray, 1991, p. 321). Ethical norms, while idealistic, are important in moving the profession in a strategic direction as a cohesive whole.

Control of Internal Competition

A key feature of professional culture relates to the implicit and explicit control of internal competition, a topic broached in Chapter Six in regard to dissemination of price and quality information to buyers. Health professions typically have engendered as part of their culture the belief that fellow members are not economic rivals. Rather, economic competition against one's fellow members is destructive to the professional community because it forces professionals to criticize each others' quality or other aspects of service. Criticisms and countercriticisms can escalate to the detriment of the combatants and other members of the professional community. Too, internal competition contributes to commercialization of the profession, which can diminish the community's market power in relationships with buyers.

Management of internal competition by the professions has typically been enacted through formal codes of ethics, formal rules in licensing laws, and informal norms communicated via peer pressure. As Berlant (1975) has described, for example, the medical profession historically used provisions within its code of ethics as a means to discourage competitive behavior between members. The "ethical" canons concerned prohibitions against advertising, bargaining, fee splitting, and contract medicine, as well as "principles" concerning fee fixing, fee discrimination, and the acceptability of third parties. Since it has been subjected to critical antitrust and legal action beginning in the 1970s, this ethical strategy has diminished as a control mechanism over intraprofessional competition.

There are, however, forces other than ethical and legal constraints that control intraprofessional competition. Evans (1980) has suggested that several factors — the existence of relatively small medical markets, shared training experiences, continuing associations in professional activity (for example, within the hospital), social relationships, and the value placed on reputation — are conditions for "conscious parallelism" among the members of a professional community. Practitioners may develop strong relationships. Withholding consultations or referrals, as well as labeling someone with a "bad" reputation, are sanctioning mechanisms. It is clear that this strategy to control competitiveness is more likely in professions with a high degree of interdependence among members — a condition most likely met by health professionals who undergo extensive training and education.

Also affecting internal competition are the size of the profession as a whole, discussed earlier in this chapter, and the size of specialties within the profession. A common dimension of internal competition is that between generalists and specialists. The dental profession has implemented norms against internal competition by requiring specialists to limit their practice to their specialty, thereby removing a competitive threat to the generalists (Feldstein, 1988b). Orthodontists, for example, must refer routine dental work to general dentists. The medical profession, unable to implement quite so controlling a strategy, settled instead for allowing specialists to perform generalist work but encouraging the practice of "board certification," as discussed in Chapter Three, to reduce the degree of overlap between the work of generalists and specialists.

The management of internal competition using these conventional mechanisms must take into account the growing demand that professionals should be accountable for the price and efficacy of their services. Without information to enable them to shop around for the most cost-effective practitioners, buyers will be unable to exert the influence they seek. Legislative, judicial, and regulatory stakeholders as well hold values that are suspicious of the self-protectionist potential of cartels of professionals. This means that many professions will need to accommodate levels of internal competition that historically they have been able to avoid.

Internal Quality Control

Another important dimension of the internal culture of a profession is the degree to which members protect each other from regulatory bodies—which relates to the greater problem of managing the quality of services given by the profession's members. The "conspiracy of silence" is powerful in many of the health professions, and it serves an important integrative function. Members of the professional community commonly share the belief that the inexact nature of their knowledge base occasionally leads to unfortunate outcomes and accommodates a wide range of opinion about appropriate professional behavior, creating a reluctance to challenge their colleagues' judgment. Practitioners may be informally sanctioned if they "rat" on their fellow practitioners. In medicine, this policy has led to widespread tolerance of mistakes (Bosk, 1979; Millman, 1977). Practitioners are expected not to testify against each other in malpractice cases, since the same untoward episodes could happen to them. Complaints filed by professionals against their peers for malpractice are relatively few—even though many states require professionals to report instances of malpractice they observe. Underpinning this pattern is the fact that licensing boards in most states are composed primarily of members of the regulated professions.

If integration of the professional community were the only concern, professional communities might ignore all but the most extreme episodes of professional misconduct—those that most practitioners agree are ethically egregious. But legitimacy and market power are threatened when buyers and regulators discover that shoddy professional practice has been shielded by members of a profession. Professional communities must therefore pursue effective internal policing of their members, and informal sanctions against poor practice, such as labeling the practitioner as "bad" and reducing referrals, should be encouraged. Professional associations typically have formal procedures for dealing with certain types of misconduct by members, and they encourage reporting of severe problems. As an example, in 1991 the American College of Healthcare Executives approved a policy on "impaired healthcare executives" stating that executives have an ethical and professional obligation to report substance abuse and mental impairment of colleagues "to the appropriate person or persons" should their colleague refuse to seek assistance (American College of Healthcare Executives, 1991).

To manage internal quality more effectively, health professions can act more quickly to embrace new technologies to assess competence and promote excellence in the work of their members. Programs to aid practitioners impaired by substance abuse are common, but these efforts assure just a minimum level of competence. To enhance legitimacy with external stakeholders and the morale of practitioners, professions could develop incentives for the "pursuit of excellence" as vigorously as they have urged the establishment of a minimum level of competence. Such incentives might include the recognition by licensing boards or professional associations of exceptional performance or perhaps the establishment of quality management teams based on industrial models.

Apart from management of its knowledge base and culture, management of a third resource of the professional community — its organization — is critical to establishing integration and strategically adapting to change. We address organizational strategies at two levels: the professional community as a whole, including all associations, and the level of the primary professional association. At one extreme, strategic decision making throughout the professional community may be centralized in one primary professional association. Although this is unlikely to happen in a large or complex profession, in any event the primary association's role is a pivotal one.

Adaptation Through Organization:
The Primary Professional Association

To overcome problems of size and differentiation and to formulate strategy on behalf of individual members, professional communities typically have established one organized entity: the primary professional association. As noted earlier and illustrated in Table 1.2 in Chapter One, all health professions have established a dominant professional association as part of the legitimating process. The association is important in representing the professional community to external stakeholders and for initially creating internal cohesion (Hofoss, 1986). A classic study by Akers and Quinney (1968) rates the following five health professions in descending order on degree of unity and integration within the professional community: dentistry, medicine, optometry, pharmacy, chiropractic. Separate rankings of the unity and integration of the primary professional association were identical to the rankings of *community* unity and integration, suggesting the importance of a strong primary association.

Primary professional associations face management issues similar to those of any voluntary organization. We discuss these issues under the headings of inclusiveness, resources, and structure of the primary association.

Inclusiveness of the Primary Association

The inclusiveness of the primary professional association is the degree to which its membership includes the whole profession. Despite the efforts of most professional associations to keep entry barriers to a minimum, many of them fail to draw widespread support. The American Medical Association has about 44 percent of the country's physicians among its membership, for instance, although some 90 percent of physicians belong to the state associations that are represented in the AMA's House of Delegates (L. Wagner, 1990). Only about 20 percent of working registered nurses belong to the American Nurses' Association (Kovner, 1990). Professional associations face the "free rider" problem: nonmembers have little incentive to join if they can enjoy the same benefits as members at no cost. Thus, to attract members, most professional associations keep dues low and market group membership benefits such as insurance policies. In the past some professions, such as occupational therapy, have required association membership as a condition of certification or licensure.

Of course, members' commitment to the association may vary considerably. As noted above, there are other sources of integration in the community, and common association membership may not be "necessary" to create close bonds among professionals. This may be the case for medicine, for example.

Resources of the Primary Association

Professional associations vary in the degree to which they are able to garner the resources necessary to pursue their goals. The budget and staff of the primary association for several different health professions are shown in Table 7.1.

Most associations have relatively small staffs and budgets: those listed in Table 7.1 average some 2.6 staff per 1,000 members and spend about $310 per member. Associations with fewer staff and financial resources include those representing dental hygienists, medical technologists, registered nurses, and radiologic technologists. Associations with greater resources include those covering health care administrators, podiatrists, and MDs. Because of the limited amounts of money that can be raised through member dues, successful professional associations have creatively expanded revenue sources beyond member dues (Martin, 1989). Thus expenditures per member typically are higher than member dues.

As with membership, more resources do not necessarily lead to more effective organizations. But resources are necessary for such activities as lobbying external stakeholders and marketing the profession — functions that are quite important in achieving legitimacy and market power. The considerable resources of the American Dental Association and American Medical Association no doubt have facilitated their success in the legislative arena (Feldstein, 1991). Many professional associations maintain Washington offices for the purpose of lobbying Congress. At least thirty-two different medical specialty associations have Washington offices (L. Wagner, 1990). The American Nurses' Association in 1990 maintained a Washington staff of twenty-six, and it sponsors its own political action committee (PAC) and has a grass-roots lobbying network of

Table 7.1. Resources of Primary Professional Associations: 1990.

Profession	Members	Staff	Budget	Staff per 1,000 Members	Budget per Member
Administrators, health care	23,000	100	$12,000,000	4.3	$522
Administrators, long-term care	6,700	20	$2,500,000	3.0	$373
Chiropractors	20,000	30	—	1.5	—
Dental hygienists	30,000	39	$4,200,000	1.3	$140
Dentists	140,000	380	$42,100,000	2.7	$301
Denturists	—	1	$40,000	—	—
Dietitians	60,000	139	$15,000,000	2.3	$250
Medical record administrators	31,000[a]	65	$6,000,000	2.1	$194
Medical technologists	20,000[a]	15	$1,900,000	0.8	$95
Nurse anesthetists	24,500	50	$9,000,000	2.0	$367
Nurse-midwives	3,000	16	$2,200,000	5.3	$733
Nurses, registered	200,000	190	$17,000,000	1.0	$85
Occupational therapists	45,000[a]	120	—	2.7	—
Optometrists	29,000[a]	100	$14,300,000	3.4	$493
Pharmacists	40,000[a]	70	—	1.8	—
Physical therapists	51,000[a]	124	$15,000,000	2.4	$294
Physician assistants	13,000	30	$3,500,000	2.3	$269
Physicians—DOs	21,700	93	$5,000,000	4.3	$230
Physicians—MDs	271,000	—	$183,500,000	—	$677
Podiatrists	9,200	46	$6,300,000	5.0	$685
Psychologists	70,000	305	—	4.4	—
Radiologic technologists	16,000	24	$1,400,000	1.5	$88
Recreational therapists	3,200	2	—	0.6	—
Respiratory therapists	30,000[a]	—	$5,900,000	—	$197
Social workers, medical[b]	134,000	200	$14,500,000	1.5	$108
Speech-language pathologists and audiologists	60,000	—	—	—	—

Note: Dash indicates data not available.

[a]"Members" include people from other affiliated occupations in addition to the one listed.

[b]Figures for medical social workers are for all social workers.

Source: Data for MDs are from Somerville, 1990, p. 43; data for others come from Burek, 1992.

Congressional District Coordinators (Hill and Hinckley, 1991). In 1991, the ANA moved its national headquarters from Kansas City to Washington. The AMA, as well, employs a Washington lobbying staff of some forty persons, and the AMA's political action committee, founded in 1961, is a perennial top five contributor to national political activities (Hill and Hinckley, 1991). In fact, five of the top six congressional PAC contributors in 1989–90 were health professional associations: the American Medical Association, American Dental Association, American Academy of Ophthalmology, American Optometric Association, and American Nurses' Association (*Health Week,* Nov. 5, 1990, p. 14). No doubt the resources of professional associations will continue to flow to key decision-making sectors in the polity. To the extent that state and local areas assume importance in setting health policies, resources should be shifted to those levels. To do so, however, requires appropriate structures.

Structure of the Primary Association

To manage geographic dispersion, primary professional associations typically are differentiated into local, state, and national units. Requirements for local, state, and national membership vary from profession to profession. Examples from several professions follow.

The American Dental Association, perhaps the most tightly coupled association at all geographic levels, requires coterminous, compulsory membership at the local, state, and national levels. The American Chiropractic Association, on the other hand, is a national organization only: there are few formal organizational ties between national and any state associations, and there are few local associations. The American Medical Association is primarily a federation of state associations, and some states (six in 1990) also require membership at the county level. The AMA has set up incentives, such as reduced dues, for state medical societies to require their members to also join the AMA (American Medical Association, 1990b). Until 1949, the AMA was largely a federation of county societies with state and national membership flowing automatically from county affiliation. County membership was crucial for most specialists, as it was required for hospital admitting privileges (Feldstein, 1988b). The AMA's House of Delegates has more than four hundred physicians who represent different geographic areas, specialties, and special interests. The American Nurses' Association is a federation of state nursing associations with national membership following automatically from state membership. Nurses join local associations, which are organized into the state associations. Delegates from the state associations meet annually at a national convention to set policy for the ANA. The federated state structure was adopted in 1982 (Hill and Hinckley, 1991).

As a management issue, associations must balance the degree of connectedness among their subunits. Too much integration creates structural rigidity, conformity, and a failure to accommodate different responses to external forces that vary from subunit to subunit. Yet a tightly coupled and centralized association is able to make decisions and implement them more quickly than a loosely coupled one.

Structure can be used to facilitate response to change. To retain a leadership role in their professional community, primary associations must be open to structural change. As noted above, several professional associations have altered their structures in recent years in response to these changing conditions. Multinational corporations have faced similar issues of structuring. Gupta and Govindarajan (1991) classify subsidiaries within multinational corporations according to the flow of information from the larger corporation to the subsidiary and vice versa. The more information required from the subsidiary, the more strategic control the subsidiary should be granted. In the same way, constituent member associations can be viewed as subsidiaries of a national association. In general, autonomy should be extended to subunits of the national association when the subunits face distinctive strategic issues. If managed care networks principally are negotiated and built on a local level, for example, then local professional associations will be key participants in those developments. State or national associations are unlikely to be as effective. To the extent that buyers and regulators aggregate at the state or national level, however, retention of power and control at those levels by professional associations is good policy.

Adaptation Through Organization:
The Professional Community

Primary associations in many health professions face an even greater challenge to their leadership — the fragmented associational structure of the professional community. The multiplicity of associations in the health professions seriously complicates the traditional role of the primary association as the voice for members of many health professions. For the professional community, the issue of managing relationships among the diverse associations is a key strategic issue.

Proliferation of Professional Associations

The individual members of a professional community can seek quite divergent goals from their community. Practitioners may wish to socialize with their peers. They may seek to influence public policy in a direction beneficial to their particular subcommunity. They may wish to advance the scientific basis of the community or that of their subcommunity. The goals of educators and researchers may diverge from those of practitioners. Given the growing size and complexity of most health professions, it is unlikely that any single organization can encompass all these diverse goals. Therefore, health professions commonly develop separate formal organizations for many of the profession's subcommunities. A variety of professional associations, accommodating policy, scientific, and social interests of members, are found in each of the larger and more complex health professions. The greater number of organizations is related to the fact that they generally are low-budget operations deriving their funding primarily from annual dues and contributions and relying on volunteer labor for much of their work.

The diversity of professional associations reflects differentiation in the internal demography of the professional community, specialization in its knowledge base, and complexity in its task environment, as different associations may deal with different key sectors or groups of external stakeholders. Examples of associations formed around personal attributes are associations that represent racial minorities — such as the National Medical Association, a physician group, or the National Dental Hygienists' Association. Practitioners in training commonly are offered special student membership within the primary professional association or in an affiliated student association. The larger professions have several subcommunity organizations based on area of specialization. Medicine has over two hundred specialty societies, some with regional, state, or local units (Brailer, 1987). Many professional communities have political fundraising organizations, or political action committees, reflecting the need to interact with stakeholders in the political sector.

Apart from differentiation by type or function, associations are differentiated by levels of geography, as noted above. Most professions have international associations, reflecting the links among the same profession in different countries. Members of the larger professions have significant interaction, formally organized or not, at the local level. Physicians are tightly organized in many local markets, for instance, with a high degree of interdependence among practitioners (Havighurst and King, 1983a, 1983b). Local unity is maintained through referral patterns, hospital staff privileges, medical society membership, and informal communications. Other professions, with smaller numbers of members in local markets, are not so differentiated by geographic level.

One obvious problem following from the proliferation of formal organizations is that it is expensive, difficult, or near-impossible to coordinate strategy at the level of the professional community as a whole. Communities with larger numbers of different associations face greater integration problems. To the extent that goals of the associations conflict, the profession cannot speak with one voice to external stakeholder organizations. In pharmacy, for instance, hospital and community pharmacy associations compete for strategic decision-making power. In nursing, the National League for Nursing historically has held significant authority in the professional community — and frequently has disagreed with the American Nurses' Association, the primary association of registered nurses. The Council of State Boards of Nursing is another powerful association in nursing whose strategies sometimes diverge from those of the American Nurses' Association (Styles, 1982). In medicine, the largest specialty organization, the 68,000-member American College of Physicians, has pushed more vigorously for national health reform than the American Medical Association.

Interorganizational Coordination

As noted in Chapter Two, strategic decision making among the associations and individuals in a professional community generally occurs in a "social choice" context: associations and individuals make decisions exclusively at the association or individual level with little or no formal control at the level of the whole collective. The profession of registered nursing, for example, does not make strategic decisions — individual nurses and their associations do. If coordination increases, decision making becomes more "coalitional" or even "federative" (Warren, 1967). In the coalitional decision-making context, individuals and associations collaborate informally for the sake of community goals without a formal community structure. Federations formalize the relationships, although decisions remain primarily at the individual and association member level.

   Professions seeking to adapt strategically will develop coordinating mechanisms that directly address processes for decision making among the multiple organizations. This requires movement along the continuum away from social choice toward the coalitional and federative models. Coordinating mechanisms can range in intensity from exchange of written communications, to direct contacts, to liaison roles in each association, to joint task forces. At the highest level of coordination, a permanent coordinating federation can be created.

   Large, complex professional communities, in particular, face critical strategic problems regarding coordination of the vast network of associations within the profession. Such problems are familiar to large business firms, particularly those that operate in global markets, due to the differences among countries (Porter, 1990). Generally, decentralization accompanied by strong coordination and communication enables a business firm to be flexible and responsive to different local or country settings. In the same way, professional communities can structure themselves as decentralized coalitions or federations of associations. This may or may not be achieved under the leadership of the primary professional association.

In recent years, the American Medical Association, for example, has faced increased differentiation within medicine based on gender (more female physicians) and salaried employment (more employed physicians). Specialty associations such as the American College of Physicians have expanded in size and significance. Such developments strain the ability of the primary association to maintain integration, resulting in assessments like the following one by a physician: "Organized medicine [the AMA] is anachronistic in today's society, not for what it is or who it represents but for its central control of the decision-making process. It will eventually be forced to open itself to the numerous stakeholders in medicine" (Brailer, 1987, p. 75). The AMA has attempted to broaden its federative role. In 1990, for example, the American College of Surgeons, with about fifty thousand members, was offered one official representative slot in the AMA's House of Delegates — among some four hundred slots, most of them allocated by geographic area. The college declined the seat (L. Wagner, 1990).

Aside from the coordination problem, there is another management issue surrounding the proliferation of formal organizations within the profession: formal organizations rarely facilitate their own demise, and organizations that do not fit the changing needs of the profession may persist well beyond their useful years. For this reason, newer professions, with fewer "inappropriate" formal organizations, may be more integrated and have structures that are more consistent with current demands. The newer professions are more likely to have a field of organizations within the profession that is more appropriate to today's environment.

A related problem is that associations may pursue their own goals and thrive on conflict rather than cooperation with other associations in the same profession, as each organization tries to maximize its influence within the professional community. An interesting example of the problem of managing diverse associations and interests is the conflict between educational program associations and practitioner associations in many health professions. If practitioners believe that a profession is oversupplied relative to demand, they are likely to support a downsizing in the number of academic programs or the number of students admitted to them. Often they are opposed by educational program associations whose members do not wish to "downsize." Dentistry recently has weathered such a conflict, for example. These conflicts may take extraordinary efforts at communication and compromise to resolve.

Interprofessional Alliances

Associations in one profession also may join with associations in other professions to form strategic alliances. In the early 1980s, for instance, the American Medical Association sponsored a collective of some 172 different organizations that produced a "Health Policy Agenda for the American People" (Hirt, 1987). The primary professional associations of health care administrators, long-term-care administrators, dentists, registered nurses, optometrists, pharmacists, podiatrists, and psychologists were among the groups participating. The resulting policy document moved the collective in the direction of jointly responding to the new environment, with many suggestions for coordinating resources across the professions. For example, a consortium of organizations was proposed to advise on supply and distribution of the health professions.

Another example is the Pew Health Professions Commission, financed by the Pew Foundation, which is devoted to contributing to a "catalytic force" that will "transcend the boundaries of the individual professions and attach itself to the synergy of working across all of the health professions" (O'Neil and Hare, 1990, p. 4). The commission has focused on identifying the changes needed to adapt professional education to society's needs. Its existence illustrates the potential for such collectives to exist. To the extent that strategic issues cross the boundaries of individual professions, and to the extent that buyers and regulators aggregate in mass, we can expect accelerated development of task forces and permanent consortia across the health professions in response.

A concrete issue that requires interprofessional cooperation is the development of cross-trained personnel and patient care teams in health care delivery. As related in Chapter Four, many services can be delivered more cost-effectively by coordinated teams of professionals rather than independently functioning individual providers. Managed care, integrated care, or coordinated care systems all rely on more extensive integration across professional boundaries. Heightening the acceptance of working together and teaching the skills of cooperation are tasks that the strategic alliances of professions can do much to facilitate.

Another neglected area for interprofessional cooperation is the creation of greater mobility among health professions. As buyers and regulators search for more cost-effective ways to deliver care and match supply and demand in different professions, pressures will mount for better-integrated systems of movement between similar professions. Cooperation with such efforts will signal the professions' responsiveness to stakeholder demands.

Globalization of Professional Communities

A final key development affecting the organization of health professional communities is globalization. The boundaries of all the health professional communities in the United States are expanding geographically. One source of internationalization is demands, both from individuals and from governments, for cross-national mobility of health practitioners. The European Economic Community (EEC, or Common Market) countries are dealing with the issue of mobility of professionals by moving toward standardization of training and quality control. A

Midwives Liaison Committee, for example, coordinates activities of the national associations of midwives in the EEC (Orzack and Calogero, 1990). The North American Free Trade Agreement of 1992 proposes similar mechanisms for enhancing the mobility of professionals between Mexico, the United States, and Canada.

Another pressure for globalization is competition from foreign countries. Global competition now influences most industries in the United States and will do so even more in the future. Suppliers, buyers, and substitutes are more and more likely to be located outside the United States. American health professions increasingly face international challenges to their market power. Examples are Japanese ascension in the area of dental patents, German advances in biotechnology, cheaper medical services available across the border in Canada, and the growing contribution of non-U.S. researchers to the knowledge base of clinical medicine (Stossel and Stossel, 1990).

The globalization of the American economy means that health professional communities in the United States increasingly will need to interact with, coordinate with, or compete against professional communities in other countries. In most professions and for most strategic issues, cooperative strategies are appropriate. Most health professionals have "brother and sister" professionals and professional associations in other countries. Few have taken advantage of the opportunity to exchange strategic ideas and develop a common culture with an eye toward a global market in personnel.

One potential vision of the future is that of global professional communities, not unlike international business firms, in which new entrants may be educated in one geographic region, distributed into practice across different regions, and monitored by international standards. The pursuit of legitimacy, market power, and internal organization and management of the professions would be global tasks. Professions already headed in that direction would have an advantage. The Association for University Programs in Health Administration (AUPHA), for example, a member association of the professional community of health administrators, has moved energetically to establish a leadership role in creating legitimacy for health administrators in Latin American countries by upgrading educational standards. AUPHA has formed affiliate associations in Canada and South America. Because the division of health labor is more refined and the educational qualifications of the health professions in the United States generally are greater than those in other countries, many U.S. health professional communities have opportunities to export their educational and research technologies to certain countries.

Moreover, U.S. health professional communities have much to learn from the experiences of their colleagues abroad. As other countries become innovators in technology and treatment, the health professional communities in the United States must be ready to take advantage of those advances. As the United States struggles with reform of its own health care system, experiences from other countries inevitably are drawn into the debate (Field, 1989; Glaser, 1991; Hollingsworth, Hage, and Hanneman, 1990), and international comparisons can help a profession create new alternative visions for its own future in the United States.

Managing the Change Process

The process of adapting to a new environment requires attitudes and behavior that recognize and accept the need for change. Management of the change process is a primary dimension of strategic adaptation.

Obstacles to Change

Change frequently is theatening to individual members and associations in the professional community — particularly those who are in powerful or rewarding positions relative to others. For professions that historically have been successful, change is particularly threatening.

Internal characteristics of professional communities make them hard to change. First, the loose coupling inherent in the professional community makes coordinated response to change difficult to achieve, favoring the status quo. Compared to the ability of a formal organization to implement change, the professional community is encumbered by its lack of centralized control. Second, a large proportion of practicing professionals are likely to have entered the profession under more benevolent conditions and through a socialization process that stressed different values than today's. This leads to a majority of "conventional" practitioners within the ranks. Additionally, earlier entrants may not possess the same knowledge base that is consistent with changing conditions. In pharmacy, for example, experienced practitioners are less likely to have received the education necessary for them to work in clinical pharmacy counseling. Yet the experienced members of a profession are more likely to have built the reputations and financial base that allow them to participate in the leadership activities of the professional community. That is, the more experienced practitioners are likely to have a greater influence on formal strategic decision making.

Related to this generational problem is another structural feature of professions. Change is difficult because professional communities are basically democratic. Strategic decisions are made in public, or become public, and they are processed over long periods of time through legitimated structures. Therefore, it is difficult to introduce changes that may be effective in the long term if they run counter to the interests of large numbers of current practitioners. Nursing's struggles with upgrading educational standards to the baccalaureate level are related to the large numbers of individual members who entered the profession with associate degrees or diplomas.

Finally, most organizations develop a "commitment to the past" due to traditions, myths, personal relationships, and self-interest (Pfeffer and Salancik, 1978). The more successful professions are particularly prone to argue that old strategies should be retained. By the same token, the less successful professions may adopt a fatalistic acceptance of their positions — which also is anathema to creating change. These professions, such as medical technology, face significant hurdles in creating a culture for change within their professional communities.

Facilitating Change

In creating an internal environment that encourages change, professional communities can learn from the experiences of organizations. Change involves education and communication. It involves commitment from top leadership but participation throughout the organization. Education requires resources and takes time. Leaders of professions often have perspectives and information not widely shared by practitioners, who devote most of their time to delivering services rather than worrying about strategy and structure of the profession. Educational programs to inform members of the changing external environment, as well as the profession's options for response, should be ongoing. For new entrants to the profession, this requires collaboration between practitioners and teachers. For veteran practitioners, there must be education through programs at professional meetings and through standard communication outlets such as professional journals.

Change usually produces loss. For many experienced health professionals, this is clearly the case: a longing for the good old days is common. When change is upsetting to more experienced members of a professional community, coopting them is a possibility. As discussed earlier, "grandfathering" — exempting currently qualified members from the need to meet new requirements — is a common strategy for coopting opposition to change. The ANA, for instance, has resolved that adoption of new educational requirements for licensure "would not jeopardize the licenses and practice rights of those licensed before the effective date of such requirements" (Carter, 1986, p. 6). Beyond cooptation, the early involvement of groups likely to resist change is likely to reduce their resistance.

If the sense of loss is widespread, it is important to create rituals of transition: "opportunities to both celebrate and mourn the past and help people evolve new structures of meaning" (Bolman and Deal, 1991, p. 401). Symbolic events such as the publication of retrospective histories, which dignify the good old days but underscore their passing, can help practitioners make the transition to the new era. Support services for disillusioned practitioners, such as early retirement planning or facilitation of continuing education, are another possibility.

Another common strategy for facilitating change is to introduce it incrementally. For example, some innovations can be tested in a few states or local areas selected for their receptiveness to new ideas or other criteria. To promote the requirement that registered nurses receive a baccalaureate degree for licensure, in 1984 the ANA House of Delegates committed financial resources to five states to support implementation of their plans (Carter, 1986). The geographic differentiation within most national associations is ideally suited for the testing and development of innovations on a small scale.

Change also requires a concentration of resources — a setting of priorities. This again is difficult for professional associations, as it is easy to disperse resources over the assorted goals and programs desired by diverse and often conflicting subcommunities. Professional associations, particularly those that strive to represent the whole profession, are likely to try to be all things to all people but end up with no major accomplishments. In this sense, Hall (1982) has written that professional associations can never be completely effective — their conflicting goals can never be satisfied. Strong leadership will be necessary to promote the setting of priorities.

Leadership Requirements

Leadership in professions typically is enacted through participation in top positions in a primary professional association or a publication distributed throughout the professional community. In medicine, for instance, Morris Fishbein, long-time editor of the *Journal of the American Medical Association,* and Arnold Relman, former editor of the *New England Journal of Medicine,* influenced the direction of the profession from those posts, while James Sammons, former executive vice president of the AMA, is an example of an influential association leader. A survey of health leaders in the mid-1980s identified Sammons as the most powerful person in health care in the United States (Brailer, 1987). More visible at the local and state level are the thousands of health profession leaders who participate in professional association committees, educational programs, regulatory boards, and local and state politicking.

Just as Porter (1990, p. 615) urges for corporate leaders, the leaders of professional communities must see their profession within a larger context — an interdependent, global one — and energize their professions "to meet competitive challenges, to serve demanding needs, and, above all, to keep progressing." New leadership of the health professions involves creating and managing change within the professional community. Leaders will need to create visions of the future and persuade others to help create that future, rather than defending the past and reacting to challenges as they evolve.

The need for change requires that leaders stimulate controversy, that debate and conflict be encouraged, and that controversial actions be taken. Turnover of old leadership is required, as well, so that new ideas can be championed. Contemporary leadership of professional associations in health care will require that leaders push their organizations to take positions that may not have broad-based support at first. Leaders more often will need to shape rather than reflect the positions of their associations. Even the leadership of the medical community, renowned for its policy conservatism, has recently changed its approach to national public policy issues, adopting a more positive and proactive stance. (See Hill and Hinckley, 1991; Koska, 1992; see also the May 1991 issue of *JAMA* on "Caring for the Uninsured and Underinsured.")

Practitioners can help their professions adapt to the changing environment by electing leaders and appointing association executives who are not afraid of change and innovation. Rather than old-guard professionals or respected academics, some associations, such as the American College of Physicians (Brailer, 1987), are turning to the managerially trained professional who is more apt to be comfortable with managing change.

A neglected aspect of the strategic adaptation process in professional communities is the assessment of performance of associations and their leaders. This requires that goals be defined and progress in meeting the goals be monitored. Leaders of professional communities often are not held accountable for their leadership performance. Instead, leadership posts may be viewed as honorific positions that reward service over many years. This is a luxury that most professions can ill afford today.

As for leaders of *subcommunities* within the profession, they must assess the role of their subcommunity within the larger context of the professional community to ensure that the professional community as a whole benefits from the subcommunity's actions. This involves reaching out to other subcommunities and often to the primary professional association. If the primary association is not the logical place to achieve such coordination, a steering committee of subcommunity association leaders might be reasonable. The dangers of disunity, or the missed opportunities that result, make it essential that leaders of the subcommunities work together.

Strategic adaptation of the profession is not just the realm of top officers in professional associations or journal editors. Because most health professionals have significant direct contact with the public, their own actions in the workplace and elsewhere affect the profession's relationship with external stakeholders. Some observers contend, for instance, that individual physicians are more influential with the American public on medical policy issues than are government and labor leaders (Blendon and Altman, 1987).

Most members of the health professions have been relatively uninvolved in the strategic activities of their professional communities. As we contend in Chapter One, most health professionals and their leaders are accustomed to an unusually high degree of trust, respect, and deference from major stakeholders in their task environment. Today, practitioners need to understand that their work world is not so secure. It is not safe just to do the work they were educated to do. Individual practitioners by definition belong to a collective organization, a professional community, that requires energy and commitment and resources from its members. If that professional community fails, the practitioner suffers. Therefore, individual practitioners should care deeply about how the professional community handles strategic challenges. They should participate in and

Table 7.2. Strategies for Internal Organization and Management.

Conventional Strategies

- Standardize entry education and internalize research organizations.
- Exempt experienced practitioners from new educational requirements.
- Strengthen the internal culture by an intensive initial socialization period and onerous postentry certification.
- Strengthen the internal culture by discouraging competition within the professional community and tolerating a conspiracy of silence.
- Rely on the primary association to represent the professional community.

Contemporary Strategies

- Devote resources to matching the supply of practitioners with market demand.
- Encourage diversity of gender, race, and ethnicity in the professional community.
- Work with external stakeholders to identify new knowledge to incorporate in entry and continuing education. Emphasize lifelong learning.
- Prepare for less control over work domain boundaries in the workplace.
- Accommodate internal competition in response to external stakeholders' demands.
- Intensify internal quality management.
- Rely on federations or coalitions across multiple associations to represent the professional community.
- Form strategic alliances with other professions to pursue common goals such as cross-training, development of patient care teams, and mobility between professions.
- Expand links with professional communities in other countries.
- Facilitate internal change by introducing it incrementally, educating and involving those who may resist it, and offering support for those who view change as a loss.
- Support leaders who are not afraid of change and innovation. Assess leadership performance and stimulate turnover in leadership if necessary.

---

shape the role of the primary association for the profession as a whole. They should assess leaders and hold them accountable for progress of the professional community.

Conventional and Contemporary Strategies

In addition to managing relationships with their buyers, suppliers, regulators, and substitutes, professions must manage relationships among the loosely coupled, internal units of the professional community. In the health care industry of the 1990s, all professions face challenges to internal organization and management. Conventionally, integration of the diverse elements of the community has been achieved through standardized entry education and socialization, internalization of new knowledge development, and an internal culture that discourages competition and encourages a conspiracy of silence. Internal organization of the professional collective has been focused on one primary professional association; a multitude of diverse associations serve less central demands of internal stakeholders.

To enhance strategic adaptation, a series of contemporary strategies is listed for consideration in Table 7.2.

Generally the strategies suggest ways that professional communities can better adapt to demands of external stakeholders, sometimes at the sacrifice of cohesion within the community. These actions include increasing the diversity of personal attributes in the profession, meeting society's needs for an adequate supply of practitioners, incorporating new knowledge (including that generated outside the profession), and expanding levels of internal competition and quality management. Moreover, cooperative alliances among associations within and among professions and the international community are warranted. These contemporary strategies require that the professional community embrace change rather than shunning it. New leadership of the professions will challenge individual members to change, and individual members will hold leaders accountable for successful strategic adaptation of the profession.

PART THREE

Profiles of Diverse
Health Professions

Chapter Eight

Meeting the Challenges:

Change and Adaptation in Five Health Professions

The guidelines for strategic adaptation developed in the previous chapters are meant to apply to most health professions. But strategies are more or less relevant to particular professions depending on the configuration of each profession's internal structure, stakeholder relationships, and environmental pressures. For professions such as psychology that do not depend much on suppliers, for example, strategies to manage relationships with suppliers obviously are less relevant. Challenges from large buyer groups affect dentistry less than medicine. Employed professionals face different strategic challenges than independent practitioners.

In this chapter we examine some of these differences, using five health professions as case examples. We comment on issues surrounding the accomplishment of legitimacy, market power, and appropriate internal organization and management of the five professions.

Assessing the strategies of professions is a subjective task, and advising professions on their future strategic direction is speculative as well as subjective. These appraisals are posed to stimulate introspection, debate, and action, as well as to demonstrate application of the strategic adaptation framework in a comparative fashion across several different professions. As the case examples are relatively brief, readers with detailed knowledge of specific professions — particularly those who are members of the professional communities being reviewed — should compare their own observations with our "external" perspectives.

Selection of Case Examples

From the twenty-six health professions listed in the tables throughout this book, we use five professions as case examples: allopathic medicine (MDs), optometry, registered nursing, physical therapy, and occupational therapy. These professions represent a wide range of variation on several dimensions. One of the case professions, allopathic medicine, has a level of market power associated only with a few other professions — osteopathic medicine and dentistry among the ones mentioned in this book. (Veterinary medicine, not covered in this book, would be included in this group as well.) In their relationships with buyers and substitutes these professions maintain substantially greater market power than other health professions. Allopathic and osteopathic medicine and dentistry have stronger and more extensive work-domain monopolies than other health professions and therefore face fewer substitute threats to their core activities. Because osteopathic and allopathic medicine have cultivated a cooperative merger strategy, their substitutability is not a strong competitive challenge to either profession. Moreover, each of these professions has a substantial proportion of self-employed members, and therefore each is less dependent on employers than the other health professions.

There are important differences among allopathic medicine, osteopathic medicine, and dentistry, of course. Through the actions of health care insurers, buyers of physician services are gaining in strategic consequence more than are buyers of dental services. Osteopathic medicine faces legitimacy issues that dentistry and allopathic medicine do not. Because allopathic medicine is the largest and most internally differentiated of the three, it faces more formidable internal organization and management problems.

Several health professions have substantial proportions of self-employed practitioners, from which significant market power relative to buyers is derived, but face more critical substitution challenges than do medicine and dentistry. These include chiropractors, optometrists, podiatrists, and psychologists. Within this group, chiropractic confronts legitimacy concerns the others do not. Podiatry is small and relatively undifferentiated, psychology large and highly differentiated. From among these professions we examine a medium-sized profession: optometry.

Dental hygiene, denturism, pharmacy, social work, most of the allied health professions, the administrative professions, and nursing are all distinguished by their market weakness relative to substitutes and strong buyers — the employers and the other professions on whom these professions depend. Registered nursing has complex and unique strategic issues due to its unusually large size and high degree of internal differentiation. In discussing registered nursing, we also comment on the position of nurse-midwives and nurse anesthetists. Physical therapy is an intriguing case because of recent dramatic accomplishments in expanding its market power. Occupational therapy has interesting contrasts to physical therapy. One other profession, pharmacy, was the subject of substantial commentary in Chapter Five due to its distinctive dependence on suppliers.

Less represented by our case examples are newer professions, such as physician assistants, and those professions whose work domain is most closely controlled or supervised by medicine or dentistry. This category would include dental hygiene, radiologic technology, and physician assistants. These communities face a greater need to establish legitimacy as professions than do the case examples. The administrative professions, including medical record, health care, and long-term-care administration, are not represented in the case examples either. Their strategies would differ somewhat due to their stronger incentives to cooperate with, indeed represent, the employer — the health care organization — in relationships with other health professions and external stakeholders of the organization.

Framework for Assessment

For each case example, we intertwine assessment of the profession's market power, legitimacy, and internal management with discussion of the strategic outlook for the professional community. Legitimacy is gauged by success in implementing such conventional strategies as credentialing, high levels of entry education, standardization of the sites of education, recognition by organized buyers, and government support for education and research. Internal organization and management issues are raised by commentary on the standardization and control of entry education, integration of teachers and researchers, strength of the initial socialization experience, and resources and membership of the primary professional association. Market power is indicated by monopolization of a work domain relative to substitutes as well as independence from powerful buyers (including employers) and powerful suppliers.

In order to discuss the strategic outlook of each profession, it is necessary to speculate on future changes in their task environments. Thus we note prominent trends in the relationships of each profession with its key suppliers, buyers, and substitutes, as well as with regulators and teachers and researchers, and suggest appropriate strategic responses to these trends.

Allopathic Medicine: From Control to Cooperation

Allopathic medicine has achieved a collective performance record that other professions seek to emulate. The profession attained strategic success through simultaneous achievement of legitimacy, market power, and strong internal organization and management in the early 1900s (Starr, 1982). Scientific medicine gave hope to millions that disease could be conquered, elevating medicine to the height of social legitimation. Market power was established by licensing laws that have been altered very little since the late 1800s, laws essentially marginalizing or banning any substitutes that are not subordinate to physicians and prohibiting the practice of medicine by non-MD corporations.

Integration of teachers and researchers was achieved by

the Flexner Report reforms in the early 1900s, which eliminated most of the for-profit academic institutions that were not interested in research. Control over entry education was consolidated by the AMA, and standardization of the curriculum was achieved. Medicine was able to differentiate into a large number of certified specialties, beginning with ophthalmology in 1917, while maintaining the basic standardized education shared by all practitioners. The primary professional association, the AMA, successfully represented its members, particularly the private solo practitioners, and was rewarded with support by the professional community. For many years, the professional community of medicine has been able to exert huge strategic leverage in relationships with other professions, legislators, and buyers by using the community's impressive level of resources to influence important issues — such as government controls over physician reimbursement and credentialing requirements for allied health and nursing professionals.

While medicine's bold undertakings in the early 1900s to integrate the suppliers of knowledge and monopolize a broad work domain clearly served it well for many decades, new challenges to the professional community are calling for new and resourceful strategic actions. Among the new strategic challenges for the medical profession, the most important considerations concern buyers. With regard to public-sector buyers, the Congressional Budget Office has predicted huge future federal budget deficits and has singled out health care entitlement programs as the major source of the problem (Starobin, 1992). If such deficits create pressure for progressively stringent reimbursement for physicians under Medicare, then a countervailing power strategy is a likely response by medicine. Its effectiveness, however, will require the creation of a unified coalition of the various professional associations in medicine — a task made more difficult by the differential effect of payment changes on different specialties.

In the private sector, too, the escalation of health care costs will pressure buyers to constrain physician reimbursement. Faced with more powerful buyer structures, physicians should respond with strategies that have a structural foundation. For employed physicians under salary pressure from hospitals, unions can provide a basis for a countervailing power strategy. In managing relationships with health plans, physicians can develop structures to pursue either a countervailing power strategy or a competition strategy, as explained in Chapter Six. Without their own structure, physicians should bridge with organized buyers by assuming influential roles in their organizations and addressing their concerns.

One must not overlook strategies concerning the general market conditions of supply and demand when considering buyers. Concerns of buyers and regulators that "too many" physicians are a source of cost escalation, that primary care physicians are undersupplied, and that inner city and rural areas are undersupplied should not go unaddressed by the professional community. Cooperation in the matching of supply to market demand is essential for maintaining medicine's legitimacy. As one medical educator observes relevant to the current system of graduate medical education, "the system responds more promptly to professionals' interests and institutions' service needs" than the health needs of the population (Martini, 1992, p. 1097). Increased responsiveness to the demands of external stakeholders is likely to require closer articulation of the undergraduate and graduate medical education systems (Mullan, 1992) and greater incentives for educational innovation (Barzansky and Gevitz, 1992).

An effective reduction in the total supply of new physicians may raise additional strategic considerations. As academic members of the medical community may resist an entry restriction strategy, a judicious bridging strategy with medical schools will be important. In addition, geographic and specialty shortages in medicine resulting from a reduction in the supply of physicians may boost the substitution challenge from other health professions willing to fill any "vacant niches." Therefore, the issues of specialty and geographic mix need to be managed concurrently.

On the demand side, medicine should support the expansion of health insurance for the uninsured. Not only will the demand for medical services increase, but the medical profession will gain greater legitimacy with the broad population for assuming this position on such a sensitive issue. It should be noted, however, that this strategy will induce further increases in health care costs and therefore exacerbate pressures from buyers. Thus it is especially critical that the profession take action to address the cost concerns of buyers.

While managing relationships with buyers poses serious strategic issues for medicine, substitutes are a less severe, but chronic, concern. First, emerging structures that combine financing and service delivery (for example, HMOs and PPOs) emphasize routinization and efficiency — thus incentives for "least-cost inputs" are strong. This logic favors replacing high-cost medical labor with lower-cost substitutes. Conventional strategic responses, such as marginalization and efforts to delegitimate substitutes, are unlikely to be effective in the new environment. Medicine should use cooperative strategies to manage relationships with substitutes in the work setting. In bureaucratic settings, the physician's prominent role will facilitate use of the relational strategies. Physicians should be prepared to accept a more cooperative and less controlling set of relationships with interdependent professions like nursing in order to meet new demands for cost control.

A second substitute pressure, mentioned earlier, arises from the undersupply of physicians in rural areas and the inner cities. If substitutes occupy these geographic niches and demonstrate their efficacy, then the conventional strategy of delegitimating substitutes with claims about their incompetence will be undercut. Such beachheads in underserved areas can develop into a base for substitutes to claim similar functions in more mainstream locations. If medicine does not take the initiative in addressing rural and inner city undersupply issues, other professions will fill the void. In that case, medicine should be prepared to accept cooperative arrangements with those professions.

A third source of challenge from substitutes is the continuing appeal of alternative healers to the public. Since the failure of conventional medicine to "cure" certain health problems is one reason for this phenomenon, evaluation of the outcomes of alternative medicine suggests certain strategic solutions. Successes can be assimilated into mainstream medicine; failures can be used to challenge the legitimacy of the alternatives. Medicine, however, must also address a "process" issue in this area. Alternative healers often are seen as caring for the holistic and spiritual nature of the patient, while the medical profession is seen as dealing with patients in a detached "scientific" manner (Frohock, 1992). One solution to this matter is greater emphasis on the importance of patient/physician interaction in the socialization and education of physicians, both at the entry level and beyond.

In addition to the substitute challenges stemming from bureaucratization, undersupplied locations, and alternative healers, two serious substitution issues may emerge in the future. First, medicine has traditionally protected itself from incursions by substitutes by developing new and more complex knowledge and techniques. If medical research investment continues to slow or decline and the current techniques and knowledge become more routinized, however, the challenge from substitutes may increase. In response, medicine must continue to seek legitimacy from society in the form of investment in medical research. Criticism stemming from the connection of rising health care costs and technology may arise, but medicine can respond by publicizing the public's ardent support of medical research ("Most People . . . ," 1992).

The second issue is related to the cost of medical technology. Callahan (1990) has argued that the control of health care costs will entail a shift in values from high-technology "curative" medicine to "caring" medicine. If this shift occurs, then professions such as nursing will become more empowered. As noted earlier, medicine must emphasize the process dimension of care and the professional community must enhance the status of medical specialties such as family practice.

Internal differentiation within medicine suggests another important strategic concern: integration within the professional community. Medicine is no longer a relatively homogeneous body of self-employed primary care practitioners. Complex biomedical knowledge has created a huge number of specialties in medicine, and with these specialties has arisen a stratified profession with divergent interests. As suggested earlier in discussing the RBRVS payment system, the internal divisions could increasingly assume a zero-sum character.

Centrifugal forces within medicine will sorely test its internal cohesion. While the influence of traditional structures such as the AMA and the county medical societies has been waning, the external challenges to medicine may reinvigorate these structures as forces for integration. Failing this development, integrative forces may shift to informal networks of physicians at the local market level and to physician groups in bureaucratic work settings. If a relatively high proportion of younger physicians continue their current employee status as they age, traditional medical associations may be challenged by unions to represent the interests of physician employees. Given the internal differentiation of the medical community, such a response may be appropriate. But maintaining a degree of collective integration in the midst of this diversity will be a major challenge for the professional community in the future.

Finally, there are two issues concerning legitimacy that should be mentioned here. First, recent criticisms of medicine — charging unnecessary and inappropriate care, the absence of systematic evaluation of the results of medical procedures, and the variation of medical standards in different locations in the country — have raised questions about the scientific character of medicine. As emphasized in Chapter Three, science remains a basic legitimizing value for medicine. Such questions therefore challenge the deference that medicine can elicit from society. With obvious concern about costs, private and public buyers have increasingly developed practice guidelines. This trend usurps a traditional function of the medical community and suggests to practitioners that the public has doubts about their competence. It is essential that the medical community, through the AMA and specialty associations and its academic subcommunity, undertake and publicize the evaluation of procedures and technology in order to maximize its control over the development of practice guidelines. Otherwise, medicine will be forced to use a countervailing power strategy in its efforts to influence the development of practice guidelines by organizations outside the medical community.

The second issue concerns the image of medicine. While technical competence rooted in scientific education is a basic factor in attaining legitimacy for physicians, the medical community must recognize that less rationalized matters are important too. Physicians have cultivated an image of "professionals" whose behavior is governed by service norms that lead them to act in the best interests of their patients. Such actions as physicians referring patients to imaging centers in which they have a financial interest, however, as well as the gaming of reimbursement processes, suggest that a "business" image of self-interest is equally accurate. If these practices become widespread, physicians risk the loss of social deference and ultimately an erosion in their legitimacy. Indeed, the business image seems to justify the trend toward treating physicians as "units of labor" subject to efficiency evaluation. The medical community faces a difficult situation — particularly because some of the untoward behavior is an outgrowth of entrepreneurial responses to the "free market" emphasis in health care. Strategically, however, the medical community must adopt and enforce a set of ethical guidelines to govern behavior in these new conditions. Otherwise it will increasingly be viewed as just another business.

Successful strategic adaptation by medicine will require a broad shift in the direction of the contemporary strategies outlined in previous chapters. This effort will require allocation of resources to educate members of the profession on the need for change. It will also require that strong leaders make unpopular decisions to push rather than follow their constituencies within the profession. These are daunting challenges for a profession that historically has been in a position to control rather than cooperate with key stakeholders.

Optometry: Strategic Choices of a Substitute Profession

Optometry emerged in the early 1900s from the occupation of refracting opticianry, and since that time the professional community has steadily gained legitimacy and market power (Begun,

1981). Optometry's identification with science and health has been undeniable, and optometrists have been licensed in all states since the first quarter of the twentieth century. As access to university settings was initially denied, optometry successfully used an independent college strategy to develop its educational base. Entry education is standardized and centrally controlled by the professional community, as four years of intensive education and socialization in optometry schools is required after at least two years of college. (Most optometry students hold a bachelor's degree.) A national code of ethics was adopted in 1944, about twenty-five years after medicine formalized its code. A strong primary professional association (the American Optometric Association), with over 75 percent membership, is a significant advantage to the professional community.

The major strategic issue confronting optometry arises from the combination of its legal marginalization and the presence of significant substitutes. While opticians cannot perform vision examinations, they sell eyeglasses and contact lenses, thus competing with optometry's dispensing function. Ophthalmologists (MDs), who have a legal monopoly on ophthalmic surgery, can perform any service also delivered by optometrists. Ophthalmologists have been a historic competitor with optometry in the area of refraction (vision examinations to determine lens needs), and while they have often left the lens dispensing function to opticians, ophthalmologists increasingly are retaining this task for themselves. A predicted oversupply of ophthalmologists in the future, if realized, will only intensify this competitive situation. Additionally, while the majority of optometrists are self-employed, there is a segment of so-called commercial optometrists within the profession. They are employed to do refractions by high-volume lens dispensers, an arrangement that further intensifies the competitiveness within the ophthalmic market. Finally, some retail drugstores and other outlets are encouraging consumers to buy eyeglasses "off-the-shelf," essentially substituting self-care for the services of vision care professionals.

Reducing its legal marginalization through diversification of its work domain is an appropriate strategy for optometry. The profession has begun this process by shifting its educational programs to a "more comprehensive, holistic approach to patient care," one that teaches students "to take a complete medical history and to understand the effects of systemic diseases on the ocular system" (Raffel, 1984, pp. 147–148). An important dimension of this broadened education is training in the use of diagnostic and therapeutic drugs. In the last two decades, optometrists have gained the legal right to use diagnostic drugs in all states and therapeutic drugs in most states, a right previously monopolized by ophthalmologists. The professional community succeeded in this strategy through judicious deployment of organizational resources at the state and legislative district level (Begun and Lippincott, 1980; Begun, Crowe, and Feldman, 1981). The strategy has been endorsed by key stakeholders, such as the American Public Health Association (1991, p. 243), which claims that "expansion of the clinical privileges of optometrists has increased the availability, accessibility, and cost-effectiveness of eye care to the American public."

The use of diagnostic and therapeutic drugs may make an important contribution to redefining optometry's legitimacy and power within the ophthalmic market. With an enhanced diagnostic capacity, optometry can better position itself as the "primary care" vision profession. This position is strengthened by the significantly lower costs of educating optometrists than ophthalmologists (Miller, 1992). Presumably, optometry could dominate initial patient contacts for vision problems and work cooperatively with ophthalmology, which would be relegated to a specialized market niche of surgery. Essentially, then, ophthalmology would become dependent on optometry through the referral process. In some managed care programs, optometry has been installed in such a gatekeeper role for vision services ("Managed Eye Care . . . , 1993).

This clearly is an ambitious strategy, and its success will be strongly influenced by optometry's continuing efforts to enhance its legitimacy vis-à-vis a high-status medical specialty. Thus it is important for optometrists to continue their efforts to gain hospital privileges. If they are successful, this would help to diminish the status advantage that ophthalmology derives from its access to hospitals.

Recognition of optometry by buyers is important as well. Gaining coverage from public and private buyers for optometric services not only enhances its legitimacy in society at large, but it also strengthens demand for the services. Medicare and Medicaid have included optometry in their coverage, but optometry currently is fighting for recognition by buyers such as HMOs and PPOs. Emphasizing its cost-effectiveness relative to ophthalmology, as well as promoting its enhanced quality stemming from changes in the educational programs, will be useful strategies for optometry in this area. A conventional strategy — pursuing legal and legislative remedies to require coverage of optometric services — is another possibility.

While a primary care role may give optometry greater market power over vision examination services, the existence of high-volume lens dispensers makes control over the dispensing function more problematic. Laws forbidding the employment of optometrists largely have been overturned, and the customer's right to the results of the vision examinations (lens prescriptions) has made the eyewear market more competitive. Optometrists have relied on conventional strategies — claiming that the services of self-employed optometrists are of higher quality, for example, and emphasizing to consumers the need for joint demand of the product (a lens) and the services of the optometrist (diagnosis, prescription, and follow-up). More promising contemporary strategies include supporting the creation of competitive conditions in the lens manufacturing industry and accommodating the increased competition that derives from segmentation of the lens prescribing and lens dispensing functions.

This analysis assumes that ophthalmic technology will stay relatively constant — possibly a tenuous assumption. Technological developments, such as laser surgery on the eye, may make the correction of vision defects possible without the need for lenses. The implications are clear. If surgery replaces lenses as the prominent method to correct vision problems, ophthalmology could virtually dominate the market because optometrists cannot perform surgery in most states. At the extreme, optometry may become obsolete if "one-stop shopping" with an ophthalmologist provides a surgical solution to diagnosed vision problems.

While laser technology may not become a widespread replacement for lenses, its potential suggests the importance of new knowledge and technology for optometry's future. The emergence of a holistic approach to patient care indicates that optometry is becoming more similar to ophthalmology. But the profession's continuing distinctiveness probably will depend on the degree to which its academic subcommunity can develop techniques and procedures for its practitioners that differ from ophthalmology's. If optometry were to expand its work domain to include types of surgery, then a merger strategy with medicine may be in its long-term future.

Advances in optometric techniques and procedures are important for a reason other than competition with ophthalmology. Optometry has two subordinate occupations: optometric technicians and optometric assistants. While this social structure may be functional for the performance of routine tasks, it could develop into a substitution challenge — particularly given trends in the demands of external stakeholders. If optometry does not develop a more complex knowledge base, these substitutes may make claims on more and more of optometry's tasks. Optometry already faces major substitution problems from ophthalmology and opticianry. It must be especially careful to manage its response to its own "allied" occupations.

A final strategic problem for optometry concerns internal structure. This problem has two aspects. First, the profession suffers from a generational cleavage that reflects differences in education. Unlike medicine, which has a professional culture that embraces advances in technology and knowledge, some older optometrists question whether the newer, holistic training is really "optometry." They see the profession as basically performing refraction and vision training functions. The cleavage ultimately will solve itself as the older practitioners leave the profession, but its existence underscores the importance of socializing practitioners into a culture that expects advances in knowledge and techniques.

A second strain arises from the split between self-employed practitioners and the "commercial" optometrists mentioned earlier. This is a delicate problem because both factions usually have received the same education. Historically, the professional association has emphasized that the employment context of "commercial" optometrists jeopardizes quality service because of the emphasis on selling lenses. In today's environment, however, external stakeholders support the competition-enhancing effects of commercial optometry. Optometry should therefore pursue strategies that respond to the demands for accessible and cost-effective care — which would entail accommodating "commercial" practice within the professional community. In fact, the commercial history of optometry could be used to the advantage of the whole profession. The professional community could embrace and build upon the positive aspects of its commercial past: the emphases on access and cost-effective delivery of care. These features are consistent with the achievement of greater market power and legitimacy in relationships with external stakeholders.

We turn next to three professions whose incumbents not only face the challenges of substitutes but are more dependent on powerful buyers of their services. Nursing is the first of these professions.

Registered Nursing: Managing a Huge and Complex Profession

Registered nurses are licensed in every state. The profession has achieved a high degree of legitimacy with the American public — although for its contribution to service and the "caring" side of health more than its identification with science. Educational requirements to become a registered nurse are not high — at least two years of postsecondary education are required — and are available from three major sources: associate degrees from community colleges, diplomas from hospital-sponsored programs, and baccalaureate degrees from colleges and universities. As hospitals still sponsor a large number of nursing schools, the professional community finds it difficult to exert control over the numbers of nurses produced. Educational program accreditation is controlled by the National League for Nursing, an entity separate from and sometimes at odds with the American

Nurses' Association (ANA). Pursuing a conventional strategy examined in Chapter Three, nursing is attempting to implement a more standardized system of postgraduate, voluntary certification under the aegis of the National Board of Nursing Specialties (now the American Board of Nursing Specialties), an alliance of several independent certifying agencies (Hartshorn, 1991).

The professional community of registered nursing faces significant strategic problems in three interrelated areas: relationships with employers, relationships with substitutes, and internal organization and management. In the first two areas, changes are creating new opportunities for nursing to apply contemporary strategies.

Historically, nursing has held little market power in relationships with employers. Employers have been able to draw upon the service orientation of nurses, the output of hospital diploma nursing schools, and the presence of substitutes (licensed practical nurses and nurse aides and assistants) to reduce their dependence on registered nurses. Moreover, the nursing community's historical ambivalence in regard to collective bargaining and its reluctance to strike vitiates a source of power relative to employers. In their efforts to control costs, employer organizations will continue to seek ways to routinize tasks and assign routine tasks to lower-level personnel. At the same time, physicians will continue to seek ways to create lower-level personnel within their own professional community, as was the case with the AMA's proposal in 1987 to create a nonnurse, bedside care worker — the registered care technician (originally termed registered care technologist) — under the direct supervision of the physician (American Medical Association, 1988). (The proposal was withdrawn in 1990 after intense opposition from nursing assocations.)

Together these pressures make it important that nurses respond to the employers' productivity concerns. The development or integration of subordinate personnel *within* the professional community of registered nursing, long desired by the community, would be a significant boon to the profession's market power in relationships with substitutes and employers. (Current subordinate personnel — licensed practical nurses and nurse ssistants and aides — are not well integrated into the registered nursing community.) Continued experimentation with staffing patterns is an area of joint interest to employers and the community.

For nurses employed in large organizations, opportunities for cooperative strategies with hospitals and other major employers are rising — due to the pressures on hospitals to control costs and the fact that nursing costs represent a considerable component of hospital costs. In this environment, proposals from nursing to improve efficiency and productivity in health care delivery organizations can increase the influence of nursing in these organizations. Recent successful efforts at achieving self-governance in the hospital setting are evidence of the potential for nursing's increased influence, as is the successful culmination in 1992 of nursing's long fight to gain representation on the Joint Commission on the Accreditation of Healthcare Organizations. If cooperation with employers is unsuccessful, the increased use of countervailing power through collective bargaining, under the aegis of both unions and the ANA, is likely.

Another area for the application of contemporary strategies is in relationships with physicians. The demarcation between the roles of physician and nurse is rapidly blurring (Gamble, 1989) — particularly for registered nurses who go on to receive a master's degree in a specialty field. The ability of nurse practitioners and other advanced-practice nurses to cost-effectively deliver services traditionally supplied by physicians is widely accepted. (See, for example, Office of Technology Assessment, 1986; Cromwell and Rosenbach, 1988; Knedle-Murray, Oakley, Wheeler, and Petersen, 1993.) Historically, registered nursing has pursued cooperative strategies in relationships with physicians, accepting close formal supervision from them and no direct reimbursement from patients. The opportunities for competitive strategies, such as direct competition with physicians in the delivery of selected services, are burgeoning, however, due to the broad knowledge base of advanced-practice nurses and the receptiveness of external stakeholders to physician substitutes. At the same time, many of the conventional strategic battles — such as the securing of direct third-party reim-

bursement and the standardization of educational curricula —
have to be fought as well.

Balancing integration and differentiation within the professional community is a critical issue for registered nursing.
Differentiation by educational preparation is a source of major
schism in the community, contributing to a low participation
rate (about 20 percent) in the primary professional association,
the ANA. Over 100 associations at the national level, and many
more at the state level, crowd the organizational field of nursing ("Directory of Nursing Organizations," 1990). The vast size
(1.6 million nurses and hundreds of associations) and differentiation of registered nursing ensure that integration of the community will continue to be difficult to accomplish. As argued
in Chapter Seven, external stakeholders today are less receptive
to conventional strategies for integration, such as standardizing
entry-level education. One conventional strategy for integration —
the development of research within the profession — shows promise, however, as much nursing research will focus on prevention
and care of society's major health problems ("Will We Follow
a National Research Agenda," 1990). The development of a
more scientific knowledge base for the profession is a complementary strategy.

The large size and differentiation of nursing suggest a
strategy for internal organization of the community as a whole:
a strengthening of the decentralized *subcommunities* within registered nursing, with less control and resource expenditure at
the total community level. Under such a strategy, nursing would
encourage its subcommunities to develop integrative mechanisms, including strong professional associations, within their
specialized work domains. Strategic issues within each of the
subcommunities differ, particularly on the dimensions of buyer
and substitute relationships. Strategic issues in nurse-midwifery,
for example, are intricately bound to developments in the structure and strategy of the medical specialty of obstetrics, as well
as the activities of lay midwives (DeVries, 1985). In nurse
anesthetics, strategic issues are connected to transitions in the
structure and strategy of the medical specialty of anesthesiology.
Locating the primary professional association at the subcom-

munity level empowers members of the subcommunity, as they enjoy the integrating effects of being in the same position relative to external stakeholders and therefore sharing the same strategic concerns.

The differentiation of nursing has promoted pockets of strength in the community. While we have listed nurse-midwives and nurse anesthetists as separate professions in several tables of this book, they also could be considered subcommunities loosely coupled to the larger community of registered nursing, since they share the basic educational credentials of registered nursing. These subcommunities (as well as nurse practitioners and clinical nurse specialists) have gained significant legitimacy and market power by offering themselves as cost-effective substitutes for physicians and other providers. (See, for example, a review by Safriet, 1992, which estimates the cost of physician education, and physician income, to be at least four times that for nurse practitioners and nurse-midwives.) The subcommunities of nurse anesthesia and nurse-midwifery have built strategic strength by developing strong primary professional associations, by responding to buyers' demands for cost-effective care, and by adopting entrepreneurial strategies such as the pursuit of direct third-party reimbursement and expansion of the work domain. Nurse-midwifery and nurse anesthesia have their own primary associations distinct from the ANA; the professional associations are active and energized (Bankert, 1989; Rooks, 1990); and each profession controls accreditation of its own educational programs (see Table 3.1 in Chapter Three).

As explained in Chapter Seven, there is still an important coordination role for the primary professional association of registered nurses or for a federation of associations. One community-wide issue that requires attention is the matching of nurse supply with demand. Chronic concerns about a nursing shortage hurt the profession when proposals arise for new substitute providers, such as the AMA's proposal for registered care technicians. Innovative strategies for matching supply and demand include creating incentives for practice in underserved settings, such as nursing homes, and job design that maximizes use of the RN's time for professional work (McKibbin, 1990).

Nurse-midwives and nurse anesthetists face critical problems in generating an adequate supply of practitioners (Rooks, 1990; National Commission on Nurse Anesthesia Education, 1990); a community-wide federation with an enhanced coordinating role could assist these subcommunities with the undersupply problem.

Another important role for a community-wide federation is the identification and nurturing of new market niches arising from shifts in demography and disease patterns. If the primary professional association, the ANA, were to adopt this role, it would need to structure itself as a conglomerate of specialty and other subcommunity associations, rather than a collective of state associations of individual nurses. Movement in this direction is indicated by structural changes adopted in 1989 by the ANA, which allowed multistate associations to join the ANA and specialty organizations to join state nurses associations (Selby, 1989).

To the extent that registered nursing can solve its internal organization problems — or at least put them aside and devote attention to creating market power and legitimacy within its subcommunities — its future is brighter than its past. Promising opportunities exist for the profession or its subcommunities to meet new demands from stakeholders and at the same time build legitimacy and market power.

Physical Therapy: Successful Adaptation

Physical and occupational therapy share portions of their work domains, and their work domains overlap those of nurses and several other health professionals, as was shown in Table 4.1 in Chapter Four. In physical therapy, however, energetic pursuit of largely conventional strategies has dramatically enhanced the market power and legitimacy of a professional community. Indeed, physical therapy is a modern-day case study in successful strategic adaptation.

Physical therapy arose in response to the need to treat veterans wounded in World War I and then served important roles in treating wounded soldiers in World War II and people struck with polio. Physical therapists are licensed in all states as a result of a licensing movement begun in the 1950s. Licensing boards are composed primarily of members of the profession. Entry education requires four (moving toward five) years of postsecondary education. In 1978 the profession established a specialty certification process. Success in the academic arena is associated with physical therapy's clear link to the scientific study of movement dysfunction. The profession has initiated its own doctoral-level educational programs in order to supply its own teachers and researchers. Physical therapy's legitimacy has been buttressed by legal and political strategies to achieve recognition from government and other third-party buyers. The profession's entry educational programs have received federal funding support, as well.

The primary professional association, the American Physical Therapy Association (APTA), has pushed assertively for raising entry standards from the baccalaureate level to the master's degree level. This movement has been pursued with relative success — despite some internal conflict as well as stiff opposition from consumer and academic representatives and powerful interest groups such as the American Hospital Association and the American Society of Allied Health Professions (MacKinnon, 1984; Institute of Medicine, 1989). It has even been suggested that a professional doctorate be established as the entry-level requirement by the year 2005 (Johnson, 1989). These developments in raising educational standards have been made more feasible by the profession's decision to withdraw from the AMA-affiliated organization (CAHEA) that accredits most allied health educational programs. CAHEA stopped accrediting physical therapy programs in 1983 (American Medical Association, 1990a), and APTA does its own accreditation of educational programs.

Despite some internal strife over the upgrading of entry education credentials, the primary professional association of physical therapists has remained strong: about 57 percent of practitioners belong to APTA. Physical therapy has developed its own subordinate personnel — physical therapy assistants — within the professional community. (The primary association for physical therapy assistants is APTA.) Internal cohesion has been aided by a relative shortage of therapists, which reduces internal competition.

Physical therapy has moved to address another major strategic weakness in its market relationships — its dependence on physicians as indirect buyers, owing to legal requirements that patients be referred by physicians. In 1982 APTA adopted the policy that physical therapy practice be independent of practitioner referral, propelling the profession toward greater independence from physicians. In a growing number of states, totaling forty by 1992, physical therapists can evaluate patients without medical referral; in twelve of these states, treatment of patients also is permitted (American Physical Therapy Association, 1992).

Physical therapists can be employed or contracted by large buyer organizations at rates below those charged by physicians. Furthermore, demand for physical therapy services has been enhanced by the physical fitness boom and the growing demand for chronic disease therapies in the elderly population. The profession has been well positioned to gain market power, and demand for physical therapists is quite high relative to supply (Institute of Medicine, 1989).

Thus favorable changes and astute strategic choices have created stronger legitimacy and market power for physical therapy. This success itself, however, presents a serious issue in internal organization and management. The temptation to rely on strategies that were successful in the past is strong in organizations — resulting in the adage that "success breeds failure" (Bedeian and Zammuto, 1991, p. 488). As new challenges face physical therapy, old response patterns may prove to be less successful. The marketplace advantage of having direct access to patients is likely to diminish as more patients enter managed care arrangements where interprofessional relations often are governed by gatekeepers. Moreover, the community must continue to supply enough practitioners to satisfy key buyers or it could invite substitution from physical therapy assistants or other providers (or other forms of intervention by buyers and regulators). A similar development could result if physical therapists push to upgrade entry educational requirements to the doctoral level—particularly if the price of their services escalates concurrently and they no longer present an attractive substitute to physicians.

Additionally, the professional community must be aware that challenges to its legitimacy can arise if its newfound power is abused. The commentary of one physical therapist (Peat, 1986, p. 103) is instructive in this regard: "How did Physical Therapy progress to the point where it was singled out as the 'hot' profession? A review of our advances in recent years would show aggressive marketing of the product. . . . In addition, our professional associations have been very successful in the public relations exercise of presenting Physical Therapy. . . . With this growth of practice and influence, has there been a corresponding growth in the scientific base? . . . The critics . . . would suggest that the primary energy, enthusiasm and motivation have very effectively advanced our clinical, economic and professional base but not our scientific core."

Challenges to the efficacy and cost-effectiveness of physical therapy services will assume greater import in the coming years, such that public relations exercises will be less successful in the strategic arena. To build on its recent achievements, physical therapy should shift its attention and resources in line with new requirements of external stakeholders by seeking knowledge base developments that are in concert with the needs of stakeholders for efficacious, cost-effective, and accessible services.

Occupational Therapy: Continuing Struggles

In contrast to physical therapy, occupational therapy has had more limited and belated success in establishing legitimacy and market power, despite their similar period of origin around World War I. As indicated in Table 3.2 in Chapter Three, occupational therapists are licensed in fewer states than physical therapists (forty versus fifty in 1990), and their drive to achieve licensure occurred some twenty years later than physical therapy's (Gritzer and Arluke, 1985). Unlike physical therapy, occupational therapy has not fought for educational program accreditation independent of the AMA's oversight. Third-party reimbursement of occupational therapy services, while growing, has lagged behind the achievements of some other professions, such as physical therapy and speech-language pathology (Gritzer and Arluke, 1985). For reimbursement of certain insured services, referral by a physician is necessary. Entry educational requirements remain at the four-year college degree level, despite some interest in raising them to the master's degree level. In general, occupational therapy has pursued less aggressive strategies than physical therapy.

The boundaries of occupational therapy's knowledge base are broad and malleable, and the relationship of the knowledge base to scientific theory is less clear than is the case with physical therapy. Only in recent years have serious attempts been initiated to define a "science of occupations" (Clark and others, 1991). As a result, occupational therapy has become less identified with medicine and less interdependent with physicians than physical therapy. In many work settings, such as school settings, occupational therapists may have very little interaction with physicians. This helps to explain why occupational therapy chose not to "rebel" against medicine as physical therapy did — the strains that derive from close substitution threats were simply not there.

Occupational therapy faces major substitution challenges. Physical therapy and occupational therapy share certain tasks: both may use ultrasound treatments, for example, and both claim expertise in the area of hand rehabilitation. Physical therapists, recreational therapists, and other therapists may provide services that affect a patient's occupation or "purposeful activity" — the claimed domain of occupational therapy. Consequently, the creation of a distinctive work domain for occupational therapy that has a scientific basis (a "science of occupations") is an important challenge for the profession in its struggles to differentiate itself from substitutes.

Occupational therapy has important strengths on the dimension of internal organization and management. An estimated 73 percent of occupational therapists belong to the primary association, the American Occupational Therapy Association (AOTA), as well as about half of the assistant-level providers, known as occupational therapy assistants (AOTA, personal communication, 1992). A private credentialing agency in the professional community, the American Occupational Therapy Certification Board, supplies postgraduate credentials to therapists and therapy assistants. Demand for occupational therapists is high relative to supply (Institute of Medicine, 1989). One negative structural feature is the differentiation of occupational therapists across employment settings, including school systems, hospitals, nursing homes, mental health facilities, and home health agencies. This variety makes it more difficult for the community to achieve consensus on standardizing educational curricula and delineating the profession's work domain.

Recent changes, however, offer opportunities to occupational therapy. If managed care services and ownership of rehabilitation service facilities by large corporations diminish the value of independent practice for therapists, the cooperative strategy practiced by occupational therapy with medicine may yet prove to be advantageous. Cooperative arrangements with related professions, such as physical and recreational therapists, allowing each profession to focus on particular market segments, also are likely to emerge in managed care and large corporate rehabilitation chain settings. The health promotion and holistic health movements are consistent with occupational therapy's focus on people's need for purposeful activity in contrast to a focus on medical disease. But the key to occupational therapy's successful adaptation will be the efficacy and cost-effectiveness of its distinctive services. To the extent that the profession can identify and provide such services, it will enhance its market power and legitimacy.

Comparisons and Contrasts

As the preceding cases reveal, appropriate strategic activity by a professional community can enhance achievement of its goals. Two of the five professions examined in this chapter — optometry and physical therapy — have made particularly striking gains in their legitimacy and market power over the years. But to the extent that their strategies were conventional, optometry and physical therapy could be at a disadvantage in the future. Adaptation can be hindered if old strategies are retained in a new environment, thus it may be even more difficult for professions like physical therapy and optometry, in contrast to occupational therapy and nursing, to adapt to their new positions in the health care marketplace. For some time medicine has been wrestling with this issue as well, seemingly hampered in its adaptation efforts by the fading hope that old strategies based on control will continue to be effective.

The cases illustrate the differential effect on the health professions of certain environmental changes. Threats to one health professional community may be opportunities to others — particularly when it comes to relationships with substitutes. If a profession's monopoly of its work domain is weakened, opportunities emerge for substitute professions to enhance their market power. We have seen this in the growing substitute power of nursing, physical therapy, and optometry for certain tasks historically claimed by physicians.

We also observe important differences in the internal structure of the health professions that have implications for their ability to manage key relationships. The smaller and less differentiated professions (optometry, physical therapy, and occupational therapy) are less impaired by internal divisions than the larger, more complex professions (medicine and registered nursing). Differences in knowledge base — its scientific basis and complexity, for example — also help explain the differential success of optometry, medicine, and physical therapy relative to occupational therapy and registered nursing. The former three professions have found it easier to link their knowledge base with science than occupational therapy and nursing.

On the other hand, certain challenges to legitimacy, market power, and internal organization and management touch all of these health professions. The primary challenge in all five professions is the widening power of the buyer to influence prices and other features of market exchanges, including the allocation of tasks to professions. We end by commenting on these current and future challenges to the health professions.

Strategic Adaptation in the Next Century

We began in Chapter One by describing the new sources of challenge for the health professions. Many of the compelling challenges to the power of professions coming from insurers, employers, government, and other stakeholders are driven by the escalation of health care costs. A correlated challenge is the declining accessibility to services that results from higher costs. It seems likely that cost containment will dominate the agenda of external stakeholders during this decade. To some degree, this new development "levels the playing field" of the health professions — physicians, nurses, occupational therapists, physical therapists, and other providers are being assessed by new criteria. Professions are less insulated from evaluation based on efficacy, cost-effectiveness, and access. They are less able to rely on tradition to justify legitimacy and market power.

There will be some surprises in store for the health care division of labor. The heightened receptiveness of state legislatures and other stakeholders to change is shown by the success of movements to achieve prescriptive authority for nurse practitioners, pharmaceutical use authority for optometrists, and direct patient access for physical therapy. The erosion of the old interprofessional ordering of health professions is symbolized by the AMA's recent decision to withdraw from its role as primary sponsor of CAHEA, the educational program accreditation body for twenty allied health programs, by the end of 1993. An AMA official viewed the development "as consistent with the evolution of the healthcare team and appropriate to the era we are entering, one which promises significant change in the delivery of health services" (Fauser, 1992, p. 2).

Professions that are able to balance their own interests with the changing and intensifying demands of external stakeholders will make the most gains in the next century. Contemporary strategies that recognize this need for balance were outlined in Tables 3.3, 4.2, 5.1, 6.1, and 7.2. Most of these strategies help professions to contribute more directly to the solving of external stakeholders' problems and thus underscore the interdependence of professions with society at large. The contemporary strategies recognize that more and more health care will be delivered in organizational and organized settings — calling for collaborative arrangements among the professions, no matter how competitive their relationships in the "open" market. Whatever direction national and state health policy takes in the 1990s in response to the cost and access crisis, the professions that can contribute to solving these problems will be advantaged in their relationships with stakeholders. Professions will need to devote resources to improving the cost-effectiveness of their services.

Beyond the current health care cost crisis and its resolution, no doubt new and unforeseen challenges await. In anticipation, health professions can learn from the experiences of recent years. They can do a better job of monitoring and responding to the demands of key stakeholders. They can take positive strategic action before solutions are thrust upon them. They can push their communities to innovate and experiment rather than defend and protect. They can evaluate the performance of their leadership. The larger and more differentiated professions can cultivate looser federations of stronger subcommunities rather than centralized control. American health professions can begin to globalize and form alliances with other professions in the pursuit of larger goals. If the health professions wish to preserve a prominent role in the new American health care system, they will need to respond to current and future challenges. Not to respond will invite a health care world in which professions are distrusted and professional work is supervised by managers and regulators.

References

Abbott, A. *The System of Professions: An Essay on the Division of Expert Labor.* Chicago: University of Chicago Press, 1988.

Abbott, P., and Wallace, C., "The Sociology of the Caring Professions: An Introduction." In P. Abbott and C. Wallace (eds.), *The Sociology of the Caring Professions.* London: Falmer Press, 1990.

Abramowitz, M. "Pushing Bush to a Market-Led Health Solution." *Washington Post,* Jan. 26, 1992, pp. H1, H6–H7.

Accrediting Commission on Education for Health Services Administration (ACEHSA). *Criteria for Accreditation.* Arlington, Va.: Accrediting Commission on Education for Health Services Administration, 1990.

Affeldt, J. E. "Voluntary Accreditation." In A. Levin (ed.), *Regulating Health Care: The Struggle for Control.* New York: Academy of Political Science, 1980.

Akers, R. L., and Quinney, R. "Differential Organization of Health Professions: A Comparative Analysis." *American Sociological Review,* 1968, *33* (1), 104–121.

Alperin, S., and Rose, L. A. *120 Careers in the Health Care Field.* (2nd ed.) Miami: U.S. Directory Service, 1989.

American College of Healthcare Executives (ACHE). "Ethical

Policy Statement: Impaired Healthcare Executives." Chicago: American College of Healthcare Executives, 1991.

American Council on Education (ACE). *1991–92 Accredited Institutions of Postsecondary Education.* Washington, D.C.: American Council on Education, 1991.

American Hospital Association (AHA). *Hospital Statistics.* (1991–92 ed.) Chicago: American Hospital Association, 1991.

American Medical Association (AMA). "Implementation of Report CC (I-87)." Chicago: American Medical Association, 1988.

American Medical Association (AMA). *Allied Health Education Directory.* (18th ed.) Chicago: American Medical Association, 1990a.

Amerian Medical Association (AMA). *AMA Policy Compendium.* Chicago: American Medical Association, 1990b.

American Physical Therapy Association (APTA). "Physical Therapy Practice Without Referral: Direct Access." Alexandria, Va.: American Physical Therapy Association, 1992.

American Public Health Association. "Access to Treatment for Eye Care by Optometrists." *American Journal of Public Health,* 1991, *81* (2), 243.

American Society for Hospital Personnel Administration (ASHPA). *Health Care Occupations: A Comprehensive Job Description Manual.* Hastings, Minn.: Regina Publications, 1985.

"Another Force to Be Reckoned With: The FTC." *Medical Economics,* Aug. 5, 1991, p. 45.

Anthony, M. F., and Crowley, M. A. "The National Practitioner Data Bank: A Catalyst for Review of the Credentialing Process." *Healthcare Executive,* 1991, *6* (2), 28–29.

Appleby, C. R. "Running Out." *HealthWeek,* Jan. 8, 1990, pp. 27–28, 32–34.

Aries, N., and Kennedy, L. "The Health Labor Force: The Effects of Change." In P. Conrad and R. Kern (eds.), *The Sociology of Health and Illness.* (2nd ed.) New York: St. Martin's Press, 1986.

Arnould, R., and Eisenstadt, D. "The Effects of Provider-Controlled Blue Shield Plans: Regulatory Options." In M. Olson (ed.), *A New Approach to the Economics of Health Care.*

Washington, D.C.: American Enterprise Institute for Public Policy Research, 1981.

Association of University Programs in Health Administration (AUPHA). *Health Services Administration Education, 1991–93.* Arlington, Va.: Association of University Programs in Health Administration, 1991.

Astley, W. G., and Brahm, R. A. "Organizational Designs for Post-Industrial Strategies: The Role of Interorganizational Collaboration." In C. C. Snow (ed.), *Strategy, Organization Design, and Human Resource Management.* Greenwich, Conn.: JAI Press, 1989.

Astley, W. G., and Van de Ven, A. H. "Central Perspectives and Debates in Organization Theory." *Administrative Science Quarterly,* 1983, *8,* 576–587.

Bacharach, S. B., Bamberger, P., and Conley, S. C. "Negotiating the 'See-Saw' of Managerial Strategy: A Resurrection of the Study of Professionals in Organization Theory." In P. S. Tolbert and S. R. Barley (eds.), *Research in the Sociology of Organizations.* Vol. 8. Greenwich, Conn.: JAI Press, 1991.

Backus, K. (ed.). *Encyclopedia of Medical Organizations and Agencies.* (3rd ed.) Detroit: Gale Research, 1990.

Bankert, M. *Watchful Care: A History of America's Nurse Anesthetists.* New York: Continuum, 1989.

Barley, S. R. "The Alignment of Technology and Structure Through Roles and Networks." *Administrative Science Quarterly,* 1990, *35* (1), 61–103.

Barzansky, B., and Gevitz, N. (eds.). *Beyond Flexner: Medical Education in the Twentieth Century.* Westport, Conn.: Greenwood Press, 1992.

Becker, E. R., and Rakich, J. S. "Hospital Union Election Activity, 1974–85." *Health Care Financing Review,* 1988, *9* (3), 59–66.

Becker, H. S., Geer, B., Hughes, E. C., and Strauss, A. L. *Boys in White: Student Culture in Medical School.* Chicago: University of Chicago Press, 1961.

Bedeian, A. G., and Zammuto, R. F. *Organizations: Theory and Design.* Chicago: Dryden, 1991.

Begun, J. W. *Professionalism and the Public Interest: Price and Quality in Optometry.* Cambridge: MIT Press, 1981.

Begun, J. W., Crowe, E. W., and Feldman, R. "Occupational Regulation in the States: A Causal Model." *Journal of Health Politics, Policy and Law,* 1981, *6* (2), 229–254.

Begun, J. W., and Feldman, R. "Policy and Research on Health Manpower Regulation: Never Too Late to Deregulate?" In R. M. Scheffler and L. F. Rossiter (eds.), *Advances in Health Economics and Health Services Research.* Vol. 11. Greenwich, Conn.: JAI Press, 1990.

Begun, J. W., and Lippincott, R. C. "The Politics of Professional Control: The Case of Optometry." In J. Roth (ed.), *Research in the Sociology of Health Care.* Vol. 1. Greenwich, Conn.: JAI Press, 1980.

Begun, J. W., and Lippincott, R. C. "The Origins and Resolution of Interoccupational Conflict." *Work and Occupations,* 1987, *14* (3), 368–386.

Beletz, E. E. "Games of Power and Politics: Trade Unions and Nurses' Rights." In R. R. Wieczorek (ed.), *Power, Politics, and Policy in Nursing.* New York: Springer, 1985.

Bergthold, L. A. *Purchasing Power in Health: Business, the State, and Health Care Politics.* New Brunswick, N.J.: Rutgers University Press, 1990.

Berlant, J. L. *Profession and Monopoly: A Study of Medicine in the United States and Great Britain.* Berkeley: University of California Press, 1975.

"Beverly Enlists Red Cross to Train Nurse Aides." *Healthweek,* Sept. 10, 1990, p. 7.

Birenbaum, A. *In the Shadow of Medicine: Remaking the Division of Labor in Health Care.* Dix Hills, N.Y.: General Hall, 1990.

Blair, J. D., and Fottler, M. D. *Challenges in Health Care Management: Strategic Perspectives for Managing Key Stakeholders.* San Francisco: Jossey-Bass, 1990.

Blayney, K. D., and Fitz, P. A. "The Allied Health Professions: A Critical Resource in the Future of Health Care." In E. H. O'Neil and D. M. Hare (eds.), *Perspectives on the Health Professions.* Durham, N.C.: Pew Health Professions Program, Duke University, 1990.

Blendon, R. J., and Altman, D. E. "Public Opinion and Health Care Costs." In C. J. Schramm (ed.), *Health Care and Its Costs.* New York: W. W. Norton, 1987.

Blendon, R. J., and others. "The Implications of the 1992 Presidential Election for Health Care Reform." *Journal of the American Medical Association,* 1992, *268* (23), 3371–3375.

Bolman, L. G., and Deal, T. E. *Reframing Organizations: Artistry, Choice, and Leadership.* San Francisco: Jossey-Bass, 1991.

Bosk, C. L. *Forgive and Remember: Managing Medical Failure.* Chicago: University of Chicago Press, 1979.

Brailer, D. "The Public-Spirited Physician." In D. B. Nash (ed.), *Future Practice Alternatives in Medicine.* New York: Igaku-Shoin, 1987.

Brown, D. "A New Look at Alternative Therapies." *Washington Post — Health,* June 23, 1992, p. 8.

Brown, M., and McCool, B. P. "Health Care Systems: Predictions for the Future." *Health Care Management Review,* 1990, *15* (3), 87–94.

Bucher, R., and Strauss, A. "Professions in Process." *American Journal of Sociology,* 1961, *66,* 325–334.

Burek, D. M. (ed.). *Encyclopedia of Associations.* (27th ed.) Vol. 1. Detroit: Gale Research, 1992.

Callahan, D. *What Kind of Life: The Limits of Medical Progress.* New York: Simon & Schuster, 1990.

Caress, B. "The Health Workforce: Bigger Pie, Smaller Pieces." In D. Kotelchuck (ed.), *Prognosis Negative: Crisis in the Health Care System.* New York: Random House, 1976.

Carpenter, E. S. *The Health Occupations Under Review: An Update on State Sunrise Activities, 1985–1987.* Lexington, Ky.: Council of State Governments, 1987.

Carter, E. W. *The 1979 Study of Credentialing in Nursing Recommendations: Where Are We Now?* Kansas City: American Nurses' Association, 1986.

Child, J., and Fulk, J. "Maintenance of Occupational Control." *Work and Occupations,* 1982, *9* (2), 155–192.

Clark, F. A., and others. "Occupational Science: Academic Innovation in the Service of Occupational Therapy's Future." *American Journal of Occupational Therapy,* 1991, *45,* 300–310.

Coddington, D. C., Keen, D. J., Moore, K. D., and Clarke, R. L. *The Crisis in Health Care.* San Francisco: Jossey-Bass, 1990.

Collins, R. *The Credential Society: An Historical Sociology of Education and Stratification.* New York: Academic Press, 1979.

Congressional Budget Office. *Economic Implications of Rising Health Care Costs.* Washington, D.C.: Congress of the United States, 1992.

Cook, K. S., Moris, P. J., and Kinne, S. "An Exchange Analysis of Emergent Occupational Groups: The Case of New Health Care Providers." In J. Roth (ed.), *Research in the Sociology of Health Care.* Vol. 2. Greenwich, Conn.: JAI Press, 1982.

Cooper, P. P., III, and Green, K. "The Impact of State Laws on Managed Care." *Health Affairs,* 1992, *10* (4), 161–169.

Council of State Governments. *Occupational and Professional Regulation in the States: A Comprehensive Compilation.* Lexington, Ky.: Council of State Governments, 1990.

Cox, C., and Foster, S. *The Costs and Benefits of Occupational Regulation.* Washington, D.C.: U.S. Federal Trade Commission, 1990.

Crenshaw, A. B. "When Others Choose." *Washington Post,* Sept. 1, 1991, pp. H1, H4.

Cromwell, J., and Rosenbach, M. L. "Reforming Anesthesia Payment Under Medicare." *Health Affairs,* 1988, *7* (4), 5–19.

Derber, C., Schwartz, W. A., and Magrass, Y. *Power in the Highest Degree: Professionals and the Rise of a New Mandarin Order.* New York: Oxford University Press, 1990.

Deveny, K. "Two Drugs That Fight Yeast Infections Spark a Big Marketing War." *Wall Street Journal,* May 6, 1991, pp. A1, A10.

DeVries, R. G. *Regulating Birth: Midwives, Medicine, and the Law.* Philadelphia: Temple University Press, 1985.

"Directory of Nursing Organizations." *American Journal of Nursing,* 1990, *90* (4), 143–151.

Dolan, A. K. "The New York State Nurses Association 1985 Proposal: Who Needs It?" *Journal of Health Politics, Policy and Law,* 1978, *2* (4), 508–530.

Dollinger, M. J. "The Evolution of Collective Strategies in Fragmented Industries." *Academy of Management Review,* 1990, *15* (2), 266–285.

Eisenberg, D. M., and others. "Unconventional Medicine in the United States." *New England Journal of Medicine,* 1993, *328* (4), 246–252.

Eisenberg, J. M. *Doctors, Decisions and the Cost of Medical Care.* Ann Arbor, Mich.: Health Administration Press, 1986.

Elzinga, A. "The Knowledge Aspect of Professionalization: The Case of Science-Based Nursing Education in Sweden." In R. Torstendahl and M. Burrage (eds.), *The Formation of Professions: Knowledge, State and Strategy.* Newbury Park, Calif.: Sage, 1990.

Evans, R. G. "Professionals and the Production Function: Can Competition Policy Improve Efficiency in the Licensed Professions?" In S. Rottenberg (ed.), *Occupational Licensure and Regulation.* Washington, D.C.: American Enterprise Institute for Public Policy Research, 1980.

Fauser, J. J. "CAHEA News Brief, November 4, 1992." Chicago: American Medical Association, 1992.

Feldman, R., and Scheffler, R. "The Union Impact on Hospital Wages and Fringe Benefits." *Industrial and Labor Relations Review,* 1982, *35* (2), 196–206.

Feldstein, P. J. *Health Care Economics.* (3rd ed.) Albany, N.Y.: Delmar, 1988a.

Feldstein, P. J. *The Politics of Health Legislation: An Economic Perspective.* Ann Arbor, Mich.: Health Administration Press, 1988b.

Feldstein, P. J. "Health Associations and the Legislative Process." In T. J. Litman and L. S. Robins (eds.), *Health Politics and Policy.* (2nd ed.) Albany, N.Y.: Delmar, 1991.

Field, M. G. (ed.). *Success and Crisis in National Health Systems: A Comparative Approach.* New York: Routledge & Kegan Paul, 1989.

Field, M. J., and Lohr, K. N. (eds.). *Guidelines for Clinical Practice: From Development to Use.* Washington, D.C.: National Academy Press, 1992.

Finkin, M. W., "Federal Reliance on Voluntary Accreditation: The Power to Recognize as the Power to Regulate." *Journal of Law and Education,* 1973, *2* (2), 339–375.

Finkin, M. W. "Reforming the Federal Relationship to Educational Accreditation." *North Carolina Law Review,* 1979, *57,* 379–413.

Fisher, G. W. "Optometry in Hospitals." *Journal of the American Optometric Association,* 1988, *59* (8), 588–589.

Freidson, E. "The Reorganization of the Medical Profession." *Medical Care Review,* 1985, *42* (1), 11–35.

Freidson, E. *Professional Powers: A Study of the Institutionalization of Formal Knowledge.* Chicago: University of Chicago Press, 1986.

Freidson, E. *Medical Work in America: Essays on Health Care.* New Haven: Yale University Press, 1989.

Freymann, J. G. "Medical Cost Containment: Preparing for the Year 2010." In J. D. McCue (ed.), *The Medical Cost-Containment Crisis: Fears, Opinions, and Facts.* Ann Arbor, Mich.: Health Administration Press, 1989.

Friedman, E. "The Uninsured: From Dilemma to Crisis." *Journal of the American Medical Association,* 1991, *265* (19), 2491–2495.

Frist, T. F., Sr., and Howard, S. H. "The Evolution of For-Profit Medical Institutions and Cost Containment." In J. D. McCue (ed.), *The Medical Cost-Containment Crisis: Fears, Opinions, and Facts.* Ann Arbor, Mich.: Health Administration Press, 1989.

Frohock, F. M. *Healing Powers: Alternative Medicine, Spiritual Communities, and the State.* Chicago: University of Chicago Press, 1992.

Galbraith, J. K. *American Capitalism: The Concept of Countervailing Power.* White Plains, N.Y.: M. E. Sharpe, 1980.

Gamble, S. W. "Changing Roles in the '90s: Will RNs Manage MDs?" *Hospitals,* Nov. 20, 1989, pp. 42–44.

Gaumer, G. L. "Regulating Health Professionals: A Review of the Empirical Literature." *Milbank Memorial Fund Quarterly/Health and Society,* 1984, *62* (3), 380–416.

Ghoshal, S., and Bartlett, C. A. "The Multinational Corporation as an Interorganizational Network." *Academy of Management Review,* 1990, *15* (4), 603–625.

Ginzberg, E. "Health Personnel: The Challenges Ahead." *Frontiers of Health Services Management,* 1990, *7* (2), 3–22.

Ginzberg, E. "Physician Supply Policies and Health Reform." *Journal of the American Medical Association,* 1992, *268* (21), 3115–3118.

Ginzberg, E., and Dutka, A. B. *The Financing of Biomedical Research.* Baltimore: Johns Hopkins University Press, 1989.

Glaser, W. A. "Designing Fee Schedules by Formulae, Politics, and Negotiations." *American Journal of Public Health,* 1990, *80* (7), 804–809.

Glaser, W. A. *Health Insurance in Practice: International Variations in Financing, Benefits, and Problems.* San Francisco: Jossey-Basss, 1991.

Glazer, S. "The New Nurse: Gaining More Clout in the Doctors' World." *Washington Post—Health,* March 24, 1992, pp. 12–15.

Goodman, D. "TMD Treatment Suit Highlights Practice Parameters Debate." *American Medical News,* June 1, 1990, pp. 2, 26.

Graddy, E. "Interest Groups or Information Asymmetry—What Determines How We Regulate Health Occupations?" Working Paper, School of Public Administration, University of Southern California, Los Angeles, 1989.

Gray, B. H. *The Profit Motive and Patient Care: The Changing Accountability of Doctors and Hospitals.* Cambridge: Harvard University Press, 1991.

Greenberg, W. *Competition, Regulation, and Rationing in Health Care.* Ann Arbor, Mich.: Health Administration Press, 1991.

Gritzer, G., and Arluke, A. *The Making of Rehabilitation: A Political Economy of Medical Specialization, 1890–1980.* Berkeley: University of California Press, 1985.

Gross, S. J. *Of Foxes and Hen Houses: Licensing and the Health Professions.* Westport, Conn.: Quorum Books, 1984.

Gupta, A. K., and Govindarajan, V. "Knowledge Flows and the Structure of Control Within Multinational Corporations." *Academy of Management Review,* 1991, *16* (4), 768–792.

Hall, R. H. "The Professions, Employed Professionals, and the Professional Association." In American Nurses' Association (ed.), *Professionalism and the Empowerment of Nursing.* Kansas City: American Nurses' Association, 1982.

Hartshorn, J. C. "A National Board for Nursing Certification." *Nursing Outlook,* 1991, *39* (5), 226–229.

Havighurst, C. C., and King, N.M.P. "Private Credentialing of Health Care Personnel: An Antitrust Perspective—Part One." *American Journal of Law and Medicine,* 1983a, *9* (2), 131–201.

Havighurst, C. C., and King, N.M.P. "Private Credentialing of Health Care Personnel: An Antitrust Perspective — Part Two." *American Journal of Law and Medicine,* 1983b, *9* (3), 263–334.

Hayes, D. M. "The Needs, Desires, and Demands of Employers and Employees for Cost-Conscious Medical Services." In J. D. McCue (ed.), *The Medical Cost-Containment Crisis: Fears, Opinions, and Facts.* Ann Arbor, Mich.: Health Administration Press, 1989.

"Health Industry High Pay Angers Citizens, Poll Finds," *Baltimore Sun,* March 31, 1993, p. 2A.

Health Insurance Association of America (HIAA). *Source Book of Health Insurance Data.* (1989 ed.) Washington, D.C.: Health Insurance Institute of America, 1989.

Heintz, D. H., and McNerney, W. J. "Outlook Bright for Provider-owned Systems." *Healthcare Executive,* 1992, *7* (4), 21–23.

Hershey, N. "Policy Issues Relevant to Independent Practice of the Health Professions." In *Independent Practice? What Is the Appropriate Level of Autonomy of Health Care Practitioners?* Proceedings of a conference called by ASAHP. Washington, D.C.: American Society of Allied Health Professions, 1987.

Hill, B. S., and Hinckley, K. A. "A Political Analysis of the Political Behavior of Health Interest Groups." In T. J. Litman and L. S. Robins (eds.), *Health Politics and Policy.* (2nd ed.) Albany, N.Y.: Delmar, 1991.

Hillman, A. L. "The Technologic Imperative." In D. B. Nash (ed.), *Future Practice Alternatives in Medicine.* New York: Igaku-Shoin, 1987.

Hirt, E. J. (ed.), *The Health Policy Agenda for the American People.* Chicago: American Medical Association, 1987.

Hofoss, D. "Health Professions: The Origin of Species." *Social Science and Medicine,* 1986, *22* (2), 201–209.

Hollingsworth, J. R., Hage, J., and Hanneman, R. A. *State Intervention in Medical Care: Consequences for Britain, France, Sweden, and the United States, 1890–1970.* Ithaca: Cornell University Press, 1990.

Hollis, D. V., and Taylor, A. L. *Social Work Education in the United States.* New York: Columbia University Press, 1951.

Hrebiniak, L. G., and Joyce, W. F. "Organizational Adaptation: Strategic Choice and Environmental Determinism." *Administrative Science Quarterly,* 1985, *30,* 336–349.

"Humana Revamps Its Staffing and Opens Three LPN Schools." *American Journal of Nursing,* 1990, *90* (2), 106, 117–118.

Illich, I. *Medical Nemesis: The Expropriation of Health.* New York: Random House, 1976.

Institute of Medicine. *Allied Health Services: Avoiding Crises.* Washington, D.C.: National Academy Press, 1989.

Jamous, H., and Peloille, B. "Professions or Self-Perpetuating Systems: Changes in the French University-Hospital System." In J. A. Jackson (ed.), *Professions and Professionalization.* London: Cambridge University Press, 1970.

Janeway, R. "The Costs of Medical Care in a Society with Changing Goals: A Longitudinal View." In J. D. McCue (ed.), *The Medical Cost-Containment Crisis: Fears, Opinions, and Facts.* Ann Arbor, Mich.: Health Administration Press, 1989.

Jarillo, J. C. "On Strategic Networks." *Strategic Management Journal,* 1988, *9,* 31–41.

Johnson, G. R. "Issues and Trends in Physical Therapy Education." In J. Mathews (ed.). *Practice Issues in Physical Therapy: Current Patterns and Future Directions.* Thorofare, N.J.: Slack, 1989.

Johnson, J., and Cawley, J. F. "Nurse Practitioners and Physician Assistants: Revenue and Reimbursement." In J. D. Moreno (ed.), *Paying the Doctor: Health Policy and Physician Reimbursement.* New York: Auburn House, 1991.

Jonas, S. "Health Manpower: With an Emphasis on Physicians." In A. R. Kovner and others, *Health Care Delivery in the United States.* (4th ed.) New York: Springer, 1990.

Jonas, S., and others. *Health Care Delivery in the United States.* (2nd ed.) New York: Springer, 1981.

Kass, D. I., and Pautler, P. A. "Physician and Medical Society Influence on Blue Shield Plans: Effects on Physician Reimbursement." In M. Olson (ed.), *A New Approach to the Economics of Health Care.* Washington, D.C.: American Enterprise Institute for Public Policy Research, 1981.

Kendall, P. L. *The Relationship Between Medical Educators and*

Medical Practitioners: Sources of Strain and Occasions for Coopera-tion. Evanston, Ill.: Association of American Medical Colleges, 1965.

Kissam, P. C. "Health Maintenance Organizations and the Role of Antitrust Law." *Duke Law Journal,* 1978, *1978* (2), 487–541.

Knedle-Murray, M. E., Oakley, D. J., Wheeler, J.R.C., and Petersen, B. A. "Production Process Substitution in Maternity Care: Issues of Cost, Quality, and Outcomes by Nurse-Midwives and Physician Providers." *Medical Care Review,* 1993, *50* (1), 81–112.

Konner, M. *Becoming a Doctor: A Journey of Initiation in Medical School.* New York: Penguin, 1987.

Koska, M. T. "Physician Groups Plan on Being a Major Factor in Reform Debate." *Hospitals,* Aug. 20, 1992, pp. 30, 32, 34.

Kosterlitz, J. "High-Wire Health Care Act." *National Journal,* June 22, 1991, pp. 1569–1570.

Kovner, C. "Nursing." In A. R. Kovner and others, *Health Care Delivery in the United States.* (4th ed.) New York: Springer, 1990.

Kraus, N., Porter, M., and Ball, P. *Managed Care: A Decade in Review 1980–1990.* Excelsior, Minn.: InterStudy, 1990.

Larson, M. S. *The Rise of Professionalism: A Sociological Analysis.* Berkeley: University of Californa Press, 1977.

Lazarus, W., Levine, E. S., and Lewin, L. S. *Competition Among Health Practitioners: The Influence of the Medical Profession on the Health Manpower Market.* Vol. 1: Executive Summary and Final Report. Washington, D.C.: U.S. Federal Trade Commission, 1981.

Levit, K. R., Lazenby, H. C., Letsch, S. W., and Cowan, C. A. "National Health Care Spending, 1989." *Health Affairs,* 1991, *10* (1), 117–130.

Liebowitz, B. L., and Meyer, D. C. "Doctors' Unions." In D. B. Nash (ed.), *Future Practice Alternatives in Medicine.* New York: Igaku-Shoin, 1987.

Light, D. W. "Toward a New Sociology of Medical Education." *Journal of Health and Social Behavior,* 1988, *29* (4), 307–322.

Light, D. W. "Professionalism as a Countervailing Power." *Journal of Health Politics, Policy and Law,* 1991a, *16* (3), 499–506.

Light, D. W. "The Restructuring of the American Health Care System." In T. J. Litman and L. S. Robins (eds.), *Health Politics and Policy.* (2nd ed.) Albany, N.Y.: Delmar, 1991b.

Longest, B. B., Jr. "A Cost-Containment Agenda for Academic Health Centers." *Hospital and Health Services Administration,* 1991, *36* (1), 77–93.

Lorentzon, M. "Professional Status and Managerial Tasks: Feminine Service Ideology in British Nursing and Social Work." In P. Abbott and C. Wallace (eds.), *The Sociology of the Caring Professions.* London: Falmer Press, 1990.

Lostetter, J. O., and Chapman, J. E. "The Participation of the United States Government in Providing Financial Support for Medical Education." *Health Policy and Education,* 1979, *1* (1), 27–65.

Ludmerer, K. M. *Learning to Heal: The Development of American Medical Education.* New York: Basic Books, 1985.

Luft, H. S. *Health Maintenance Organizations.* New Brunswick, N.J.: Transaction Books, 1987.

Luke, R. D. "Local Hospital Systems: Forerunners of Regional Systems?" *Frontiers of Health Services Management,* 1992, *9* (2), 3–51.

Luke, R. D., and Begun, J. W. "Industry Distinctiveness: Implications for Strategic Management in Health Care Organizations." *Journal of Health Administration Education,* 1987, *5* (3), 387–405.

Luke, R. D., Begun, J. W., and Pointer, D. D. "Quasi Firms: Strategic Interorganizational Forms in the Health Care Industry." *Academy of Management Review,* 1989, *14* (1), 9–19.

McKibbin, R. C. *The Nursing Shortage and the 1990s: Realities and Remedies.* Kansas City: American Nurses' Association, 1990.

MacKinnon, J. L. "Review of the Postbaccalaureate Degree for Professional Entry into Physical Therapy." *Physical Therapy,* 1984, *64* (6), 938–942.

McLaughlin, C. P., and Kaluzny, A. D. "Total Quality Management in Health: Making It Work." *Health Care Management Review,* 1990, *15* (3), 7–14.

McTernan, E. J., and Leiken, A. M. "A Pyramid Model of Health Manpower in the 1980s." *Journal of Health Politics, Policy and Law,* 1982, *6* (4), 739–751.

"Managed Eye Care: It's Working in Maryland." *InSight Focus,* Jan. 1, 1993, pp. 1–4.

Martin, J. "Professional Associations: A Powerful Influence on People and Institutions." In G. L. Filerman (ed.), *A Future of Consequence: The Manager's Role in Health Services.* Arlington, Va.: Association of University Programs in Health Administration, 1989.

Martini, C.J.M. "Graduate Medical Education in the Changing Environment of Medicine." *Journal of the American Medical Association,* 1992, *268* (9), 1097–1105.

Maykovich, M. K. *Medical Sociology.* Sherman Oaks, Calif.: Alfred, 1980.

Miles, R. E., and Snow, C. C. *Organizational Strategy, Structure, and Process.* New York: McGraw-Hill, 1978.

Miller, S. C. "What Is the Proper Integration of Optometry and Ophthalmology?" *Journal of the American Optometric Association,* 1992, *63* (12), 830–832.

Millman, M. *The Unkindest Cut: Life in the Backrooms of Medicine.* New York: Morrow Quill Paperbacks, 1977.

Ministry of Health, Ontario. *Striking a New Balance: A Blueprint for the Regulation of Ontario's Health Professions.* Toronto: Ministry of Health, 1989.

Ministry of Health, Ontario. *"Fact Sheet: Regulated Health Professions Act, 1991."* Toronto: Ministry of Health, 1991.

Moore, T. G. "The Purpose of Licensing." *Journal of Law and Economics,* 1961, *4,* 93–117.

Morganstein, W. M. "Auxiliary Personnel in Dentistry: An Epoch of Turf, Trends, and Territoriality." *American Journal of Hospital Pharmacy,* 1989, *46* (3), 507–514.

Moscovice, I. "Health Care Personnel." In S. J. Williams and P. R. Torrens (eds.), *Introduction to Health Services.* (2nd ed.) New York: Wiley, 1984.

"Most People Want More Medical Research." *Washington Post— Health,* July 14, 1992, p. 5.

Mullan, F. "Missing: A National Medical Manpower Policy." *Milbank Quarterly,* 1992, *70* (2), 381–386.

Murphy, R. "Proletarianization or Bureaucratization: The Fall of the Professional?" In R. Torstendahl and M. Burrage (eds.), *The Formation of Professions: Knowledge, State and Strategy.* Newbury Park, Calif.: Sage, 1990.

Nash, D. B. (ed.). *Future Practice Alternatives in Medicine.* New York: Igaku-Shoin, 1987.

National Center for Health Statistics. *Health, United States, 1990.* DHHS Pub. (PHS), 91-1232. Washington, D.C.: U.S. Government Printing Office, 1991.

National Commission for Health Certifying Agencies (NCHCA). *Sourcebook on Health Occupations.* (2nd ed.) Washington, D.C.: National Commission for Health Certifying Agencies, 1986.

National Commission on Nurse Anesthesia Education (NCNAE). "The Report of the National Commission on Nurse Anesthesia Education: Executive Summary." *Journal of the American Association of Nurse Anesthetists,* 1990, *58* (5), 384–388.

Neuhauser, D. "American College of Healthcare Executives Code of Ethics." In A. R. Kovner and D. Neuhauser (eds.), *Health Services Management: Readings and Commentary.* (4th ed.) Ann Arbor, Mich.: Health Administration Press, 1990.

Office of Technology Assessment (OTA), U.S. Congress. *Nurse Practitioners, Physician Assistants, and Certified Nurse-Midwives: A Policy Analysis.* Washington, D.C.: U.S. Government Printing Office, 1986.

Ogrod, E. S., and Doherty, R. B. "Enhanced Reimbursement Is Becoming a Reality." *Consultant,* 1988, *28* (6), 89–95.

O'Neil, E. H., and Hare, D. M. (eds.). *Perspectives on the Health Professions.* Durham, N.C.: Pew Health Professions Commission, 1990.

"Opinion Study Shows Need to Improve Administrator's Public Image." *Health Care Strategic Management,* 1991, *9* (2), 7.

Orton, J. D., and Weick, K. E. "Loosely Coupled Systems: A Reconceptualization." *Academy of Management Review,* 1990, *15* (2), 203–223.

Orzack, L. H., and Calogero, C. "Midwives, Societal Variation, and Diplomatic Discourse in the European Community." *Current Research on Occupations and Professions,* 1990, *5,* 43–69.

Pastemack, A. "Salary Row Costs HMO Exec His Job." *Healthweek News,* Dec. 2, 1991, p. 3.

Pauly, M. V. "Is Medical Care Different? Old Questions, New

Answers." *Journal of Health Politics, Policy and Law,* 1988, *13* (2), 227–237.

Peat, M. "Editorial." *Physiotherapy Practice,* 1986, *2,* 103.

Perry, S., and Pillar, B. "A National Policy for Health Care Technology Assessment." *Medical Care Review,* 1990, *47* (4), 401–417.

Pfeffer, J., and Salancik, G. R. *The External Control of Organizations: A Resource Dependence Perspective.* New York: HarperCollins, 1978.

Pointer, D. D., Luke, R. D., and Brown, G. D. "Health Administration Education at a Turning Point: Revolution, Alignment, Issues." *Journal of Health Administration Education,* 1986, *4* (3), 423–436.

Porter, M. E. *Competitive Strategy: Techniques for Analyzing Industries and Competitors.* New York: Free Press, 1980.

Porter, M. E. *The Competitive Advantage of Nations.* New York: Free Press, 1990.

Powell, T. C. "Organizational Alignment as Competitive Advantage." *Strategic Management Journal,* 1992, *13* (2), 119–134.

Powell, W. W. "Hybrid Organizational Arrangements: New Form or Transitional Development?" In G. R. Carroll and D. Vogel (eds.), *Organizational Approaches to Strategy.* Cambridge, Mass.: Ballinger, 1987.

Prospective Payment Assessment Commission (ProPAC). *Medicare Prospective Payment and the American Health Care System.* Report to Congress, June 1990. Washington, D.C.: Prospective Payment Assessment Commission, 1990.

Raffel, M. W. *The U.S. Health System.* New York: Wiley, 1984.

Reinhardt, U. E. *Physician Productivity and the Demand for Health Manpower.* Cambridge, Mass.: Ballinger, 1974.

Reinhardt, U. E. "The Compensation of Physicians: Approaches Used in Foreign Countries." *Quality Review Bulletin,* 1985, *11* (12), 366–377.

Rich, S. "Battle Over Revised Schedule for Medicare Fees Escalates." *Washington Post,* Sept. 9, 1991, p. 2.

Richardson, W. C. "Education and the Health Professions for the Next Generation." *Journal of Health Administration Education,* 1991, *9* (4), 525–540.

Ritzer, G. *Working: Conflict and Change.* (2nd ed.) Englewood Cliffs, N.J.: Prentice-Hall, 1977.

Ritzer, G., and Walczak, D. "Rationalization and the Deprofessionalization of Physicians." *Social Forces,* 1988, *67* (1), 1–21.

Roback, G., Randolph, L., and Seidman, B. *Physician Characteristics and Distribution in the U.S.* (1990 ed.) Chicago: American Medical Association, 1990.

Roberts, S. J. "Oppressed Group Behavior: Implications for Nursing." *Advances in Nursing Science,* 1983, *5* (4), 21–30.

Rodwin, M. A. "The Organized American Medical Profession's Response to Financial Conflicts of Interest: 1890–1992." *Milbank Quarterly,* 1992, *70* (4), 703–741.

Rooks, J. P. "Nurse-Midwifery: The Window Is Wide Open." *American Journal of Nursing,* 1990, *90* (12), 30–36.

Rundle, R. L. "Doctors Who Oppose the Spread of HMOs Are Losing Their Fight." *Wall Street Journal,* Oct. 6, 1987, pp. 1, 22.

Safriet, B. J. "Health Care Dollars and Regulatory Sense: The Role of Advanced Practice Nursing." *Yale Journal on Regulation,* 1992, *9* (2), 417–488.

Schieber, G. J., Poullier, J., and Greenwald, L. M. "U.S. Health Expenditure Performance: An International Comparison and Data Update." *Health Care Financing Review,* 1992, *13* (4), 1–87.

Scott, W. R. *Organizations: Rational, Natural, and Open Systems.* (3rd ed.) Englewood Cliffs, N.J.: Prentice-Hall, 1992.

Scott, W. R., and Lammers, J. C. "Trends in Occupations and Organizations in the Medical Care and Mental Health Sectors." *Medical Care Review,* 1985, *42* (1), 37–76.

Scott, W. R., and Meyer, J. W. "The Organization of Societal Sectors: Propositions and Early Evidence." In W. W. Powell and P. J. DiMaggio (eds.), *The New Institutionalism in Organizational Analysis.* Chicago: University of Chicago Press, 1991.

Seidel, L. F., Seavey, J. W., and Lewis, R.J.A. *Strategic Management for Healthcare Organizations.* Owings Mills, Md.: National Health Publishing, 1989.

Selby, T. L. "House Adopts New Structure for ANA." *American Nurse,* 1989, *21* (6), 1, 16.

Shortell, S. M., Morrison, E. M., and Friedman, B. *Strategic Choices for America's Hospitals: Managing Change in Turbulent Times.* San Francisco: Jossey-Bass, 1990.

Shugars, D. A., O'Neil, E. H., and Bader, J. D. (eds.). *Healthy America: Practitioners for 2005.* Durham, N.C.: Pew Health Professions Commission, 1991.

Sibeon, Roger. "Social Work Knowledge, Social Actors, and De-Professionalization." In P. Abbott and C. Wallace (eds.), *The Sociology of the Caring Professions.* London: Falmer Press, 1990.

Sloan, F. A., and Steinwald, B. *Hospital Labor Markets: Analysis of Wages and Work Force Composition.* Lexington, Mass.: Lexington Books, 1980.

Smith, K. R., Miller, M., and Golladay, F. L. "An Analysis of the Optimal Use of Inputs in Production of Medical Services." *Journal of Human Resources,* 1972, *7,* 208–224.

Somerville, J. "AMA Scores Legislative Victories on Medicare Issues." *American Medical News,* Jan. 5, 1990, p. 43.

Sorkin, A. L. "Some Economic Aspects of Pharmacy Manpower." *American Journal of Hospital Pharmacy,* 1989, *46* (3), 527–533.

Stanfield, P. S. *Introduction to the Health Professions.* Boston: Jones & Bartlett, 1990.

Starobin, P. "Time to Get Real." *National Journal,* Dec. 19, 1992, pp. 2874–2882.

Starr, P. *The Social Transformation of American Medicine.* New York: Basic Books, 1982.

"State Investigates Antitrust Charge Against Optometrists in Contact Lens Replacement." *Professional Licensing Report,* 1992, *5* (1), 1, 4–5.

Stossel, T. P., and Stossel, S. C. "Declining American Representation in Leading Clinical-Research Journals." *New England Journal of Medicine,* 1990, *322* (11), 739–742.

"Study to Probe Relation Between Credential and Patient Outcomes." *Professional Licensing Report,* 1990, *3* (2), 7.

Styles, M. M. "Society and Nursing: The New Professionalism." In American Nurses' Association (ed.), *Professionalism and the Empowerment of Nursing.* Kansas City: American Nurses' Association, 1982.

Toner, R. "Clinton's Health Care Plan: A Push to Sell Peace of Mind." *New York Times,* April 7, 1993, pp. A1, A21.

Torstendahl, R. "Introduction: Promotion and Strategies of Knowledge-Based Groups." In R. Torstendahl and M. Burrage (eds.). *The Formation of Professions: Knowledge, State and Strategy.* Newbury Park, Calif.: Sage, 1990.

Ulrich, D., and Lake, D. "Organizational Capability: Creating Competitive Advantage." *Academy of Management Executive,* 1991, *5* (1), 77-92.

U.S. Bureau of the Census. *Statistical Abstract of the United States: 1991.* Washington, D.C.: U.S. Government Printing Office, 1991.

U.S. Bureau of Labor Statistics. *Employment and Earnings, January 1991.* Vol. 38, no. 1. Washington, D.C.: U.S. Government Printing Office, 1991.

U.S. Department of Commerce. *U.S. Industrial Outlook.* Washington, D.C.: U.S. Government Printing Office, 1990.

U.S. Department of Health, Education, and Welfare (DHEW). *Report on Licensure and Related Health Personnel Credentialing.* DHEW Pub. (HSM) 72-11. Washington, D.C.: U.S. Government Printing Office, 1971.

U.S. Department of Health, Education, and Welfare (DHEW). *The Supply of Health Manpower: 1970 Profiles and Projections to 1990.* DHEW Pub. (HRA) 75-38. Washington, D.C.: U.S. Government Printing Office, 1974.

U.S. Department of Health, Education, and Welfare (DHEW). *A Proposal for Credentialing Health Manpower.* Washington, D.C.: U.S. Government Printing Office, 1976.

U.S. Department of Health, Education, and Welfare (DHEW). *Credentialing Health Manpower.* DHEW Pub. (OS) 77-50057. Washington, D.C.: U.S. Government Printing Office, 1977a.

U.S. Department of Health, Education, and Welfare (DHEW). *Health Resources Statistics: Health Manpower and Health Facilities.* (1976-77 ed.) Washington, D.C.: U.S. Government Printing Office, 1977b.

U.S. Department of Health and Human Services (DHHS). *Supply of Manpower in Selected Health Occupations: 1950-1990.* DHHS Pub. (HRA) 80-35. Washington, D.C.: U.S. Government Printing Office, 1980.

U.S. Department of Health and Human Services (DHHS). *Sixth Report to the President and Congress on the Status of Health Personnel in the United States.* DHHS Pub. HRS-P-OD-88-1. Washington, D.C.: U.S. Government Printing Office, 1988.

U.S. Department of Health and Human Services (DHHS). *Seventh Report to the President and Congress on the Status of Health Personnel in the United States.* DHHS Pub. HRS-P-OD-90-3. Washington, D.C.: U.S. Government Printing Office, 1990.

U.S. Department of Health and Human Services (DHHS). *Report to Congress: Progress of Research on Outcomes of Health Care Services and Procedures.* AHCPR Pub. 91-0004. Springfield, Va.: National Technical Information Service, 1991.

U.S. Department of Health and Human Services (DHHS). *Health, United States, 1992 and Healthy People 2000 Review.* DHHS Pub. (PHS), 93-1232. Washington, D.C.: U.S. Government Printing Office, 1993.

Van Maanen, J., and Barley, S. R. "Occupational Communities: Culture and Control in Organizations." In B. M. Staw and L. L. Cummings (eds.), *Research in Organizational Behavior.* Vol. 6. Greenwich, Conn.: JAI Press, 1984.

Vaughan, D. G., Fottler, M. D., Bamberg, R., and Blayney, K. D. "Utilization and Management of Multiskilled Health Practitioners in U.S. Hospitals." *Hospital and Health Services Administration,* 1991, *36* (3), 397–419.

Wagner, L. "AMA Struggles to Shepherd Diverse Flock." *Modern Healthcare,* July 23, 1990, pp. 34, 37.

Wagner, M. "Hospitals Changing Their Buying Habits." *Modern Healthcare,* Nov. 26, 1990, pp. 27–34.

Wallis, C. "Why New Age Medicine Is Catching On." *Time,* Nov. 4, 1991, pp. 68–76.

Wardwell, W. "Chiropractors: Challengers of Medical Domination." In J. Roth (ed.) *Research in the Sociology of Health Care.* Vol. 2. Greenwich, Conn.: JAI Press, 1982.

Wardwell, W. *Chiropractic: History and Evolution of a New Profession.* St. Louis: Mosby, 1992.

Warren, R. L. "The Interorganizational Field as a Focus for Investigation." *Administrative Science Quarterly,* 1967, *12,* 396–419.

"Will We Follow a National Research Agenda?" *American Journal of Nursing,* 1990, *90* (10), 63.

Wilson, F. A., and Neuhauser, D. *Health Services in the United States.* (2nd ed.) Cambridge, Mass.: Ballinger, 1985.

Witz, A. *Professions and Patriarchy.* London: Routledge, 1992.

Wohl, S. "The Medical-Industrial Complex: Another View of the Influence of Business on Medical Care." In J. D. McCue (ed.), *The Medical Cost-Containment Crisis: Fears, Opinions, and Facts.* Ann Arbor, Mich.: Health Administration Press, 1989.

Wolinsky, F. D. *The Sociology of Health.* Belmont, Calif.: Wadsworth, 1988.

Young, S. D. *The Rule of Experts: Occupational Licensing in America.* Washington, D.C.: Cato Institute, 1987.

Zimmerman, M., Dowdal, T., Hultgren, R., and Stepek, M. *Physician Incentive Payments by Prepaid Health Plans Could Lower Quality of Care.* Washington, D.C.: U.S. General Accounting Office, 1988.

Zuckerman, H., and Kaluzny, A. D. "Strategic Alliances in Health Care: The Challenges of Cooperation." *Frontiers of Health Services Management,* 1991, *7* (3), 3–23.

Index